Kristina-Downing Orr is a leading Harley Street psychologist, best-selling author and respected broadcaster. Born in Boston, she has lived, studied and worked in the UK since 1986. She was educated at Oxford, Cambridge, London and Birmingham universities and counts two doctorates among her six degrees.

A venerated researcher, she has devised two innovative psycho-therapeutic programmes, promoting personal fulfilment and happiness. In addition to her ground-breaking work in chronic fatigue syndrome, she has also reshaped treatment practices for depression and eating disorders.

She is also a playwright, with work staged in Stratford, Oxford, India and Los Angeles. She recently gave up practice to write full time. Her other works include *Rethinking Depression: Why Current Treatments Fail* (Springer, 1998) and *Alienation and Social Support* (Avebury, 1996).

Readers must consult with their doctor before deciding to make any new changes to their healthcare regime or following the advice given here. No book should ever serve as a substitute for working with a medical professional. Furthermore, because this guide is written in general terms, and since cases of Chronic Fatigue Syndrome can vary so enormously, it cannot take account of individual cases. Readers must, therefore, take full responsibility for their healthcare and any decisions made on the basis of this book's contents. While I have striven to ensure that all material here is up to date and accurate, this book is not intended to be an exhaustive review of the scientific literature available.

BEATING CHRONIC FATIGUE

Your step-by-step guide
to complete recovery

DR KRISTINA
DOWNING-ORR

piatkus

PIATKUS

First published in Great Britain in 2010 by Piatkus
Reprinted 2011 (twice), 2012
This paperback edition published in 2012 by Piatkus

A CIP catalogue record for this book
is available from the British Library.

ISBN 978-0-7499-4093-5

Text design by Sam Charrington Design
Typeset in Utopia by M Rules
Printed and bound by
CPI Group (UK) Ltd, Croydon, CR0 4YY

Papers used by Piatkus are from well-managed forests
and other responsible sources.

MIX
Paper from
responsible sources
FSC® C104740

Piatkus
An imprint of
Little, Brown Book Group
100 Victoria Embankment
London EC4Y 0DY

An Hachette UK Company
www.hachette.co.uk

www.piatkus.co.uk

Contents

APPENDICES

Acknowledgements

Many people have helped me with this project and it is to them I offer my utmost gratitude: Alan Brooke for his charm, sense of humour and early support of the book and the generous, insightful and cheerful Piatkus editors, Gill Bailey, Denise Dwyer and Claudia Dyer, with whom it has been a joy to work. Plaudits also go to Nick Clark, my typist, whose ability to decipher my illegible handwriting deserves a special award, Lesh Lender of the OMEGA group and my fellow CFS sufferers who kindly offered their time, despite limited energy, to assist me in my research. I also appreciate the generosity of Farid Monibi, Jack Kreindler, Alessandro Ferretti and Jules Cattell of the 76 Harley Street Clinic, London, once and future colleagues, as well as the support of Dr Charles Shepherd. I would also like to thank the designer, Britt Lintner, for her contribution to this project. Anne Newman, my copy-editor, also deserves special merit for her sharp eye and attention to detail. My thanks also go to Rebecca Woods for thoroughness and helpful comments.

My greatest plaudits and most humble thanks are reserved for Dr David Mason Brown and AJD who were with me every step of the way. Words can never convey my appreciation and it is to them that I dedicate this book.

Meet the Experts

The success of this programme is not only predicated on the revolutionary insights into the illness, which themselves are the product of extensive research, but also upon the qualifications and experience of the respective experts involved. All the experts here, myself (psychologist), Dr David Mason Brown (medical doctor), Alessandro Ferretti and Jules Cattell (nutritionists) are not only highly regarded professionals with decades of experience, we also work to push forward the boundaries of scientific research and work tirelessly to improve the treatments of CFS sufferers.

Dr Kristina Downing-Orr (Psychological Method)

I am a clinical psychologist, research psychologist, author, NLP practitioner, hypnotherapist, and former CFS sufferer. My background is unique from most other professionals working with CFS patients and it is this unusual combination of expertise and experience that provides the basis of this exciting new treatment approach. My first-hand experience of the devastating symptoms of the disorder, coupled with my expertise as a mental-health practitioner has enabled me to critique the medical and psychological treatments for CFS, challenge the limits of the current psychotherapeutic treatment options available and develop new, better-informed and more effective approaches. I want to promote the highest standards of knowledge, research and treatment methods possible and, most of all, protect patients from the inadequate (and often harmful) practices that are so often pushed their way. My psychological therapy reflects my extensive research and is designed specifically to motivate you and keep you focused on your goal: recovery.

Dr David Mason Brown (Medical Approach)

My research led me to Dr David Mason Brown very early on. He became my medical tutor and guide throughout my recovery process, and this book represents, in the main, a collaboration of our two areas of expertise and a mutual understanding of the illness and experiences of CFS.

An Edinburgh University medical graduate, Dr Mason Brown is a venerated and revolutionary GP. He, like me, had suffered with CFS, and it was his encounters with the limits of standard treatments that prompted him to research the illness. He is not only a practitioner, but has also been an active campaigner in improving treatments for CFS sufferers for nearly two decades. Not only has he, until recently, devoted his time as the honorary medical officer for his local CFS support group (MESH), he has also been involved in addressing the All-Party Parliamentary Group on ME set up to improve the lives of sufferers.

Dr Mason Brown's interest in CFS began when he developed the disorder and was forced to retire early from his thriving career as a GP; his symptoms were so severe that he simply could not carry on with his work. Unwilling to accept a debilitated life, however, and dissatisfied with the traditional psychological treatments on offer, he began investigating the illness. And, based on pioneering North American research of such notable vanguards as Dr Jay Goldstein and Dr Byron Hyde, Dr Mason Brown developed his own treatment protocol. His knowledge of CFS is extensive. No other physician I have ever come across in the field has demonstrated his high degree of expertise. He is not only skilled, but is also generous with his talents and works tirelessly on behalf of sufferers. His highly effective treatment protocol (the focus of Chapter Six) is designed for you to follow at home. Based on two decades of medical practice, Dr Mason Brown has found that about 80 per cent of his patients either recover completely or achieve a near-full recovery.[1]

Alessandro Ferretti and Jules Cattell (Nutritional Approach)

My research has also led me to Alessandro Ferretti (Alex) and Jules Cattell who are highly regarded nutritionists. They are both graduates of the Institute for Optimum Nutrition and co-founders of Equilibrium, a health-consulting company dedicated to advising individuals and organisations on the benefits of good health through nutritious food.

Both Jules and Alex specialise in treating CFS and are advocates for improving the lives of sufferers through more effective treatments and better-informed methods. They, like David Mason Brown and myself, are pioneers, who view the condition as a biological illness. Research and investigations that Jules has conducted on the illness provide the basis for the treatment offered here. Alex too is highly regarded in his field and has been nominated for two prestigious CAM awards. Both experts regularly give talks and lectures on a whole spectrum of nutritional issues. Their working team consists of a doctor and other healthcare professionals who combine medicine and naturopathic approaches in patient-care delivery. Based on their clinical experience, Alex and Jules report that 85 per cent of their patients will achieve near-full recovery.[2] However, although like the medical method, the nutritional approach is designed for you to follow at home, Alex and Jules recommend that you work one-on-one with a qualified nutritionist for added support.

Foreword

It is a privilege for me to write the foreword to this book. Kristina Downing-Orr's experience of CFS/ME took her on a journey from being so ill that she could only stand beside her bed for nine seconds before collapsing to a full recovery to the extent that she now walks nine miles a day.

The fact that she is also a very experienced clinical psychologist adds another dimension to her journey and – as a result – to this book, because she discovered more and more information and insights along the way which need to be shared with patients and their families and medical professionals alike. It was also a journey into the understanding of group perceptions and beliefs, some of which help, while others retard progress, and the discovery of the scientific knowledge that had been available in Canada and the USA since 1992 and built on since.

A burning desire to recover, along with the firm belief that she was actually able to do so were vital assets to Kristina. I only had the privilege of acting as a catalyst with support at a distance through emails and telephone calls, assisting in finding what worked for her. It helped also that she did not hold the common belief of some patients that they cannot get better and of many doctors that there is no cure – or even that CFS/ME does not exist!

Ignorance is not bliss. It is just ignorance. Generally speaking, we all do the best with what we know. But sadly, in areas of medicine where there is ignorance, the people who really suffer are the patients and their families. Hopefully, Kristina's insights into the causes and treatment of CFS will redress this and motivate others to become aware of other areas that may need to be tackled, including viral infections, malabsorption, nutritional deficiency, bacteria-producing toxins and environmental pollutants, to name a few.

Now it is time for Dr Kristina Downing-Orr to tell her story –

how she managed her journey to recovery and what she learned along the way – and to impart her invaluable advice to others now embarking on journeys of their own.

Dr David Mason Brown MB ChB

Although the world is full of suffering, it is full also of the overcoming of it.

HELEN KELLER

SECTION I
INTRODUCING
CFS

Introduction

The worst thing about ME [also known as CFS] is, obviously, having ME. It is spending three years in your bedroom looking at the walls, in pain, isolated, unable to read, write anything down or talk, because your brain is like spaghetti. The worst thing is having a brain which no longer works and which you can't do anything about. It's like being in solitary confinement, except you haven't done anything wrong.
JOHN (in *Shattered: Life with M.E.*, Lynn Michell)

In all the years I have been working with and researching the illness, Chronic Fatigue Syndrome (CFS) – also called Myalgic Encephalomyelitis (ME), Post-Viral Syndrome (PVS), Chronic Fatigue and Immune Dysfunction Syndrome (CFIDS), Post-Viral Fatigue Syndrome (PVFS) and Neurasthenia – I have never come across a description which better encapsulates the severity of the symptoms and the sheer depth of suffering than John's reflections above. As his haunting words convey, CFS is a debilitating illness, which destroys lives. While the numbers of those afflicted are huge, CFS remains a lonely business. And, as John reveals, it is also physically painful, cognitively demanding and emotionally devastating.

Before the onset of their condition, most CFS sufferers are active, busy people, leading full and rich lives. Once in the grip of CFS, however, they become mere shadows of their former selves, their bodies behaving like the enemy, with every waking moment a physical, emotional and cognitive struggle to function on even the most basic of levels. Many sufferers are left bedridden and housebound.

Unfortunately, despite the level of debilitation caused by CFS, conventional medicine currently offers little help, the disorder being blighted both by social stigma and a lack of professional expertise on the subject. Through my pioneering research and that of the other experts I have consulted with here, as well as my own personal experiences, I can confidently say that these short-comings stem from the failure on the part of many health professionals to recognise the true biological nature of the illness (although psychological factors do also play a substantial role in the precipitation and perpetuation of symptoms). According to researchers, despite the fact that the vast majority of people develop the condition following a viral infection[1] – in other words a *medical* trigger – sufferers are very likely to be told that their symptoms are 'psychosomatic' – or imaginary (although changes were made in 2009 to this diagnostic status with the Royal College of General Practitioners and the illness is now offi-cially recognised as medical). Despite these changes, however, patients are still usually told that depression is the root cause of their symptoms, with antidepressants and psychotherapy being the main treatment options offered. That is, of course, if a patient is 'fortunate' enough to see a doctor who recognises CFS as a genuine affliction in the first place; many physicians prefer to dismiss sufferers as attention-seekers, hypochondriacs or malin-gerers. What's more – and, as a psychologist I find this fact particularly disturbing – when patients dare to protest that their symptoms are both genuine and medical in nature, according to Gelder and his colleagues, doctors are instead routinely instructed to dismiss these claims as further evidence of neurotic disturbance.[2] In other words, they are pointed firmly in the direc-tion of the psychologist's couch.

One would be naturally forgiven for thinking that, given the psychological emphasis on the causes and perpetuating factors of CFS, the medical profession would have every confidence that psychotherapy and antidepressants would cure the affliction. However, it is officially recognised by doctors that the long-term recovery for CFS is poor because the methods used have *not* been proven to be effective.[3]

But medical professionals are not the only ones to blame. Psychologists, too, have jumped on the psychosomatic band-wagon, insisting that CFS sufferers have a fear of fatigue, leading to avoidance of activities which might increase their exhaustion.[4] This fear is exacerbated, they argue, by a consequent deconditioning of the muscles and reduced fitness, leading to increased exercise refusal. This, in turn, continues the avoidance of activity for fear of increased exhaustion. And so the cycle of psychologically induced ill health continues, they argue. Although there is an element of truth here, these are, in fact, normal reactions to chronic-disease states in which the body suffers true debilitation – often for weeks, days or months – following even the smallest exertion. Even in my profession's recent news periodical, the *Psychologist*,[5] concerns have been raised about the lack of evidence in support of the psychologically based fear/exercise-avoidant models. However, any such criticisms remain largely ignored.

So the situation is doubly tragic: with so many CFS patients feeling that they have to 'put up and shut up' for fear that they could be refused future help, they are not only ultimately abandoned and left to cope with their unbearable symptoms on their own, they also often fail to regain their health. It is the case that some patients do recover of their own accord or with limited or no intervention. However, quality of life for many is so diminished that they fall prey to any snake-oil salesman who promises to deliver a cure (causing both their health and their bank accounts to suffer), while for others, suicide can seem like the only option.[6]

My Story

I suffered from CFS following two viruses and was in the grip of the worst aspects of the illness for about two years, in no fit state to go anywhere or do anything. At some points, I was so blighted by it that I was paralysed, bedridden and barely able to function.

During that time, I had many odd aches and pains that seemed to have no obvious connection and to defy all medical logic. I was exhausted all the time and, not just that 'I'll-sit-down-for-twenty-minutes-with-a-cup-of-tea' kind of fatigue either. The exhaustion would keep going. It seemed bottomless. Then there were the migraine headaches which were blindingly painful, not to mention the visual disturbances; I couldn't see very well, particularly out of my right eye, and found bright, flickering lights particularly bothersome. My legs were as weak as jelly and would jerk uncontrollably at night, my upper arms ached with an unrelenting soreness. I would also feel faint and pass out for no apparent reason – and with no warning, either. And then, on top of everything else, I developed food allergies. My body seemed to be shutting down, although no one could tell me exactly why.

I remember being afraid of going to sleep at night, fearful, anxious that I would not have the strength to get out of bed the next morning – which was, of course, what eventually happened. I remember endless stretches of time, filled with fear, wondering if I'd ever be able to step outside or go for a walk again.

Little did I know back then that CFS would come to dominate my life. But, it did. Even now, when I feel so well and am enjoying more energy and better health than I ever thought possible, I cannot completely forget those bleak times when there was so little hope of recovery. But, that is in the past now. And, by reading my book and following my guidance, your own battle with CFS can become a memory for you too.

Millions of people around the world suffer from CFS[7] and, therefore, it has been the subject of highly specialised, but limited, academic interest. Yet respected, venerated researchers still somehow seem to draw a blank. Finding a cure for an illness is hard enough when you are well; I can assure you it's damned near impossible when you're in the throes of debilitation. But, in fact, being unable to see or walk, being so fatigued I could barely function and suffering from endless pain provided me with the best possible motivation for finding the path to recovery.

For me, there were three main incentives that forced me to realise I would have to find a cure myself: the medical profession seemed incapable of giving me the help I needed; I was still a youngish woman at the time my illness struck and there was no way I was going to spend the rest of my life as a 'viral vegetable' or 'breathing corpse'; and probably the biggest incentive was a phone conversation I had with another CFS sufferer when I first suspected I had the illness. She told me in frank, but horrific, detail about her current life and my inevitable future. She'd been suffering from CFS for several years, and although very kind and supportive, her pleasant manner could not conceal the brutal truth that was her daily existence: she'd been unable to work for years, following a virus; her social life was severely limited to the occasional brief visit of about half an hour or so with friends, but only every once in a while; and she was constantly exhausted, achy, prone to picking up viruses. She would doze during the day and yet feel wired at night and the slightest exertion would worsen symptoms the next day and trigger a decline for a week, maybe longer. She was on antidepressants to cope with the misery of such reduced circumstances and to help her sleep.

As I listened to the description of this sufferer's horrifying symptoms and the sheer narrowness of her twilight existence, my heart sank. I probed, tentatively, about the treatments on offer, but she was dismissive of them all. She'd been through the standard medical and psychological treatments, as well as a number of alternative methods, such as food-allergy therapy, but nothing had worked. She had undergone a humiliating ritual of visits to medical practitioners, often barely able to move, only to be insulted by doctors and psychologists alike, who refused to accept her illness as genuine. In fact, the local CFS consultant told her all she needed was a hobby.

When I hung up the phone I was shell-shocked. My future had been spelled out in the coldest terms – and it was no future at all. But somehow this fuelled in me a determination to find a cure and recovery. No way was I going to end up bedridden and housebound. A life half-lived was no life at all. My mantra became 'I refuse': I refused to be treated with contempt by the doctors, I refused to accept the pain and debilitation and I refused to accept my life was essentially over.

My motivation was never in doubt, but finding a cure for an incurable illness is difficult, to say the least. Ignoring the many obstacles, however, I examined my symptoms and worked out the reasons why available treatment strategies were not only ineffective in fighting CFS, but in many cases, as the evidence will show, actually made many people with CFS worse.[8] I analysed the immediate triggers of my symptoms, assessed what made me better and what made my symptoms more severe. I also spoke to twenty or so other CFS sufferers and to doctors and other psychologists who, outside their consulting rooms, would frankly admit to me that the much-vaunted psychological treatments were not as effective as patients are led to believe – something I had already suspected.

With the severely limited time and rapidly dwindling energy levels available to me, I pursued every line of enquiry. I doggedly followed every lead, no matter how vague. I became the Lieutenant Columbo of CFS, always asking, 'Just one more thing . . .' My persistence did eventually pay off though. I am well again, I've got my life back. And so could you.

How I Can Help You

By reading this book thoroughly – and you *must* do this – you can regain your health and vitality and do all those things you thought were a distant or impossible dream. Learn from my experience and my expertise. I work with the best professionals who understand CFS and are deeply concerned by the futile methods currently used to treat it. They, like me, are devoting their professional lives to improving the standard of CFS treatment.

This book will equip you with a thorough understanding of the key aspects of CFS, including its causes, giving you a greater knowledge of the condition you are dealing with. My analysis is not just the 'same old, same old', but a pioneering presentation of the latest discoveries regarding CFS, which will make clear the reasons why current orthodox methods have failed to improve your condition and may even have worsened it.

The first part of the book is mainly informative, as I believe that ignorance can play no part in a recovery programme. Knowledge is power – your first step to recovery. With the essential background facts and figures at your fingertips we will then move on to the medical, nutritional and psychological methods that will help you with your recovery: the Fusion Model.

Introducing the Fusion Model

My programme for treating CFS is based on the innovative new approach known as the Fusion Model, so called because it unites three different areas of expertise – the medical, the nutritional and the psychological – to address the different symptoms of the illness and to promote recovery.

The main objective of the Fusion Model is to first replenish the body through a choice of two options – either the medical or the nutritional – which are designed for you to follow independently at home. Although there is considerable overlap between these approaches, you are given the choice because one method might better suit your needs and lifestyle than the other. Many people with CFS have moderate or mild symptoms and do not feel the need (or desire) for prescription medication. Furthermore, some people might also feel reluctant to adopt the strong feedback-monitoring role required by the medical approach, in which case the nutritional model may be more suitable for them. In any event, remember you choose only one, and follow the instructions carefully.

The second objective of the Fusion Model is to build up psychological fortitude. Whether you are working with the medical or the nutritional approach, it is essential that you also develop psychological hardiness to tackle the stressors that are likely to have contributed to your illness in the first place and most certainly to have reinforced the cycle of ill health ever since.

Evidence in Support of the Fusion Model

The main evidence for the approaches that compose the Fusion Model comes in the form of clinical expertise and many years' experience of working with CFS patients. This has enabled close observation of the condition's development over a long period of time, including the monitoring and analysis of progress and recovery through active involvement in patients' care.

In research terms, unfortunately, CFS is not 'sexy'. It is a 'Cinderella' illness, meaning that it is an underfunded and poorly resourced area. Also, even when CFS researchers do obtain vital research grants, the vast majority favour studying the psychological treatments, shunning the biological factors that underpin the illness.

Although CFS is an affliction that affects many, the fact that cases can vary so enormously in terms of the type and severity of symptoms makes carrying out effective research even more challenging. However, my own experiences with elements of the Fusion Model, as well as Dr Mason Brown's and those of our patients are a testament to the efficacy of the programme.

Freud developed many of his theories based on his patient Anna O.; Piaget developed his understanding of childhood by mainly observing his own small brood; neuropsychologists have gained huge insights into memory deficits based on the patient HM, who was unable to form new memories following brain surgery. In a similar vein, Dr Mason Brown and I became our own research instruments, leading to the important discoveries that form the basis of the Fusion Model.

Ultimately, the decision to pursue the Fusion Model has to be yours and yours alone, but the high-quality information in these pages will help you to reach an informed decision and, should you choose to pursue it, a richer and healthier future.

How to Use This Book

While this book can be used by professionals and carers, either as a source of information or as the basis for treatment, it is mainly aimed at the CFS sufferer. Teaching you about CFS and how to treat the illness is my job. But, you have a job too.

In the first instance, you must previously have obtained a diagnosis of CFS from your doctor and consulted with him or her before embarking on this programme or making any changes to your healthcare regime. And, although the Fusion Model is designed for you to follow at home, I would advise you to work with your doctor and regularly update him or her on your progress.

Also, you must be thoroughly au fait with my views on CFS. This illness is a minefield of contentious debates between professionals, and the treatments I present here, although groundbreaking and scientifically robust, represent the minority medical view. In fact, by the time you have finished reading this book, you will, in all likelihood, be much better informed than your doctor or psychologist on the subject.

Furthermore, you will need to apply the information in the book to your own personal experiences of CFS and your symptoms. Also, you must take full responsibility for your recovery. Ultimately, no one else can do it for you – not your doctor, nor any other healthcare professional.

Having said that, however, it is truly exciting to be, finally, in charge of your own health and find yourself on the road to recovery after such a devastating illness. What's more, in terms of general recovery, there is a growing body of research showing that those people who take charge in this way are precisely those who regain their health.[9] Conversely, the 'good' patient, the compliant individual so favoured by the doctors, tends not to fare so well.

Recovery with this programme can, like the condition itself, be unpredictable. For some people it could take some time, depending upon the severity of symptoms, while for others it may be much quicker. However, in all cases there should be a steady improvement along the way.

Throughout the book, I use quotes from two women who have undergone the Fusion Model. In their own words, Marguerite and Julia, whose names and certain details have been changed for confidentiality, provide you with a helpful insight into both the illness and their recovery from it.

We – myself and my colleagues – are on your side, and we demonstrate in these pages that recovery is not only possible, but achievable. I can't even begin to describe my joy when I walked outside for the first time, having been ill for so long. Even the most ordinary things in life – ordering a curry, getting a haircut, walking in the park – became sources of great happiness for me. They still are. And they can be for you too.

> **Marguerite**
>
> After so many months of being bullied by doctors and written off as a complete hypochondriac, it was a relief to find a doctor and a psychologist who believed in my symptoms and had worked hard themselves to overcome the illness. That alone gave me confidence and inspired me to get better.

> **Julia**
>
> People with CFS, well we are not stupid. We know the difference between a medical illness and a psychological one. Thankfully, these professionals also understand that. If your doctors believe you that's 99 per cent of the battle. I got my life back. I'm well. I'm happy. And I wouldn't be able to say this without this treatment.

CHAPTER ONE
The Basics of CFS

This chapter will provide you with all the basics about Chronic Fatigue Syndrome. This is important since CFS can be difficult to diagnose and is sometimes mistaken for other medical illnesses. So the more you know, the more you will understand the nature of your symptoms. Also, because CFS is an area saturated with so much misinformation and even prejudice, your doctors might not be fully informed of the facts themselves. And, if they are not, *you* really need to be. After all, your recovery is your own personal challenge and responsibility. So the more information you have, the quicker you can recover and regain your life.

What is Chronic Fatigue Syndrome?

Let's begin our discussion of CFS by defining precisely what we mean by it.

One of the best definitions of the disorder is: 'a syndrome affecting the nervous system, immune and many other systems and organs, resulting in chronic exhaustion and/or numerous other potentially debilitating symptoms'.[1] I would further add here, that because of excessive physical or psychological strain, the body essentially 'short-circuits' and is unable to recover, leaving the person effectively in a state of permanent or semi-permanent ill-health. Accordingly, I tend to call CFS: total or near-total physical and psychological body breakdown syndrome, while David Mason Brown refers to it as potential total psychological and physiological deterioration syndrome.[2] Because the very healing mechanisms in the body break down and malfunction, they need to be fixed. In its simplest form, this is what CFS is all about: the body's inability to recover following a biological or psychological trigger.

Here are some important facts about CFS and its treatment:

- CFS is a genuine medical illness.[3] It is not a figment of your imagination. It is not synonymous with depression, nor is it a pathological need for sympathy or attention or a fear of fatigue.

- CFS is essentially a biological illness, although psychological factors do also often play a central triggering and perpetuating role. In many cases, stress both produces the onset and continuation of the symptoms. Furthermore, emotional symptoms, such as depression, can also co-exist, either due to chemical changes in the brain as symptomatic of the medical illness or as a response to a sharp deterioration in quality of life.

- The illness is plagued with myths and misconceptions and there are few medical or psychological specialists who truly understand the nature of the disorder.

- Mood disorders can also exist entirely independently of CFS.

- Problems with CFS treatments stem mainly from the fact that there is no definitive diagnostic test and symptoms are so diverse. In order to recover from CFS, you need to treat biological symptoms, learn effective stress-coping strategies and deal with any psychological factors that caused symptoms in the first place. Once the body has appropriately and sufficiently healed, then and only then do you consider reconditioning muscles and improving fitness and stamina through an appropriate exercise regime.

How Many CFS Sufferers Are There?

While CFS, to anyone who has it, can often seem like a lonely and isolated business, the condition is more common than many people think. It is not an easy disorder to quantify, however, because diagnostic standards vary enormously. So, exact figures are hard to come by. However, it has been estimated that up to 250,000 people in the UK have CFS.[4] However, Professor Basant Puri, a specialist in the field, based at Hammersmith Hospital, London, suggests that as many as 750,000 to 1,500,000 British people might meet or nearly meet the diagnostic criteria for CFS.[5]

Professor Puri further writes that in the United States there could be as many as 9 million people with the disorder,[6] although others report that 80 per cent of people with CFS never obtain a diagnosis.[7] This means there are potentially millions of others walking around with symptoms for which they receive no treatment or supervision.

As more and more research into the area is conducted and CFS gains further legitimacy, the true numbers of people afflicted will become clearer. Two things remain certain however: while the statistics might seem muddled, the illness is not so rare and you are not alone.

Who Gets CFS?

CFS can affect pretty much anyone. No one is immune. Elizabeth Barrett Browning and Florence Nightingale have both been said to have had the illness, as well as celebrities such as Hollywood director Blake Edwards and Cher.

Age

Although the stereotype CFS patient is a middle-aged female,[8] even young children and the elderly have come down with it. However, it would seem that there is mostly a thirty-year age span in early to mid-adulthood during which people are most prone to the condition. Some studies suggest that people in their teens and mid-forties are particularly likely to contract the illness.[9] But age alone is no real indicator.

Gender

Many studies show that women are more susceptible to CFS.[10] Some researchers claim females are *twice* as likely, while others argue that they are up to *four* times more likely to develop CFS compared to their male counterparts.

So women do seem to be particularly vulnerable, but why? While we still do not know the answer to this for sure, here are some credible explanations:

- Hormonal differences between men and women could be the culprit. In fact, pubescent and perimenopausal (the period of declining fertility prior to the onset of menopause) women seem to show particular susceptibility, while pregnant women sometimes report an improvement in symptoms.

- Women tend to spend more time with young children who are often carriers of infection. The teaching and nursing professions – both of which are dominated by women who spend time with children – also show higher rates of CFS compared with others.

- Women are often in charge of domestic duties and have childcare responsibilities and cannot afford the 'luxury' of rest and recuperation when ill. The added stress, both physical and mental, often worsens the situation.

- Women are much more frequently in contact with medical clinics than men (again, through childcare responsibilities) and, perhaps, are more likely to report such symptoms to doctors and to ask for help.

- Immunological differences, linked to CFS, have been noted between the sexes.

- Childbirth is a rare trigger. Although experts do not fully understand the reasons why, CFS is often triggered by extreme strain on the body. Childbirth can be both physically and psychologically traumatic and, as a result, can place excessive pressure on the woman.

- Women are often responsible for looking after ageing parents as well as children, the stress of which can be overwhelming. Again stress is a known trigger of CFS, particularly when it is unrelenting, and can lead to a weakening of the body.

While women do seem to figure highly in the statistics, a potential diagnosis of CFS in men cannot be excluded. So don't assume that because you are a man you are immune to CFS.

Personality

The medical and perhaps even the mainstream image of the typical CFS sufferer is someone with a driven, high-powered, perfectionist personality – hence the condition's early 1980s' tag of 'yuppie flu'. In fact, so-called perfectionism is often not only cited as the reason why people become ill in the first place, but also as the main stumbling block to recovery. However, this classification is a baseless stereotype, nothing more. People with all kinds of personality traits are susceptible to CFS.

Social class

Although CFS has a reputation for being associated with business executives, the condition has been found in people across the whole socioeconomic spectrum. Whether you are a prince or a pauper, CFS does not discriminate.

Genetic predisposition

Many people with CFS have been told that their illness is the product of an overactive imagination. However, research carried out in 2007 at London University by Dr Jonathan Kerr and his team[11] found that there are several genetic differences located in the immune cells (white blood cells) of people with the disorder, compared with their healthy counterparts. Although much more research needs to be conducted in this area, this is great news in terms of validating the condition. Dr Kerr's and his colleagues' discovery could possibly lead one day to a definitive diagnostic blood test. It also means that a biological foundation has been firmly established – so no more unjust accusations of malingering or hypochondria!

We've now covered the basic facts around CFS. Next, we will be looking at the symptoms of CFS and the related diagnostic criteria.

> **Marguerite**
>
> It is not possible to praise your doctors enough when they have given you your health back, especially with something like ME or CFS or whatever label it is given. You put up with so many years of abuse and unsympathetic doctors. No one believes that you are ill. You are called lazy or, worse, negative and you do your best to struggle. It was such a relief – a huge relief – when I found out that this illness was genuine. For me, that was 98 per cent of the battle. It is not very nice being called a liar or a malingerer, but I got my health back, I am no longer an invalid and I am finally well.

> **Julia**
>
> I had these symptoms for about ten years, after I got glandular fever. I was never really well after that and I never thought I would fully recover. What was worse though was that I was always depressed. I tried antidepressants, even therapy, but nothing ever really worked. I struggled to cope and pushed myself to carry on because I was expected to, but I was so tired, so miserable. Life was not worth living, I got that depressed. When I got the diagnosis of CFS, finally from Dr David

Mason Brown – the right diagnosis finally – all my symptoms began to clear up, one by one: the brain fog, the forgetfulness, even the depression. I see so many people with CFS who suffer, and they continue like that sometimes for decades. The sad thing is, they have just been following their doctors' advice because that is what you are supposed to do.

CHAPTER TWO

Diagnosing CFS

When talking about their symptoms, just about everyone with CFS, I am sure, follows the 'PDD' principle – that is, *pretty damned dreadful*. But just because you think you might have CFS, it doesn't mean you actually do. You might, in fact, have other underlying conditions or illnesses because the symptoms of CFS, particularly fatigue, are common to many disorders. As I said earlier, there is to date no definitive diagnostic test to confirm or rule out CFS and so a diagnosis is currently made on the basis of:

- A set of symptoms
- The 'six-month rule'
- Possibly some laboratory medical investigations to rule out other illnesses

Diagnostic Criteria

The first step to finding out whether or not you have CFS is to check if your symptoms meet the official requirements for the illness. I have included here two main sets of diagnostic criteria. They are very different, reflecting the continuing debates, conflicts and theoretical disputes about the illness. Have a look at both. Do your symptoms meet the criteria?

1. The Centers for Disease Control (CDC) criteria

The CDC Criteria are probably those most often used in a diagnostic setting, which is why I have presented them first. As you can see, they merely describe different symptoms, rather than making specific reference to any underlying cause. This is important, because many illnesses in addition to CFS can show similar patterns of symptomatology. In Atlanta, USA, in the late 1980s (and updated in 1994), the CDC set about defining specific symptoms relating to CFS only as follows:

Chronic Fatigue Syndrome is a disorder in which fatigue:

1. Is not medically caused by another condition
2. Is of recent onset
3. Has been evident for six months
4. Is not caused by excessive exertion (such as rigorous gym workouts or too many responsibilities)
5. Is not alleviated by resting
6. Is producing a considerable decrease in a person's work, leisure, and educational commitments

In addition, there must also be at least four more additional symptoms:

1. Cognitive impairment, including memory problems and lapses in concentration
2. Sore throat
3. Sore or tender glands (neck and armpits)
4. New or more severe form of headaches
5. Painful muscles
6. Sleep that fails to refresh
7. Post-exertional symptoms which last for more than a day
8. Painful joints, not characterised by swelling or redness

2. Canadian criteria

This is the most recent set of diagnostic criteria (see Carruthers and van de Sande, 2005[1]) and represents my professional preference for diagnosis because of its extensive symptom diversity and greater breadth of knowledge about the illness. It is also fast proving more popular in North America and its symptom specifications are now becoming recognised as the standard diagnostic tool in Europe and Australia too. The increasing popularity of the Canadian criteria reflects the growing understanding that CFS is a biological illness.

The following four symptoms must be evident to meet the Canadian criteria – how well do these reflect your circumstances?

1. Muscle fatigue and malaise following exertion, in which the recovery period can exceed twenty-four hours

2. Poor quality of sleep and feeling unrefreshed upon waking

3. Soreness of joints and muscles, headaches, nerve pain and neck aches; pain doesn't always have to be fixed – it can be migratory (i.e. move around)

4. Brain disturbances, with at least two of the following areas of dysfunction:

    • Ataxia (unco-ordinated muscles)
    • Orientation difficulties
    • Sensory and perceptual problems
    • Temporary dyslexia (problems with word recognition)
    • Cognitive impairments, including problems with word names, taking in information, categorising information, short-term memory disturbances
    • Impaired ability to concentrate and feelings of confusion

In addition to the above compulsory requirements, the Canadian criteria also include other specifications. Therefore, you must also have at least one symptom from two of the following groups (if you have any queries about any of these, it always best to speak to your doctor for clarification):

a) Autonomic disturbances

- Breathing problems
- Poor circulation
- Palpitations
- Bladder symptoms
- Intestinal symptoms
- Pallid complexion
- Dizziness or feeling light-headed
- Nausea
- Vertigo
- Balance problems
- Low blood pressure in the brain
- Rapid heartbeat
- Racing pulse
- Delayed hypotension (low blood pressure)

b) Neuroendocrine (hormones)

- Fluctuating body temperature
- Extreme sensitivity to hot and cold
- Pathological appetite, including anorexia
- Weight gain or loss
- Hypoglycaemia (low blood sugar)
- Difficulties tolerating stress
- Stress-related symptoms (anxiety or panic, for example)
- Exacerbation with delayed recovery (relapsed)
- Emotional lability (distress)

c) Immune manifestations

- Sore lymph glands
- Sore throat
- Flu-like disturbance

- All-over malaise
- Onset of new allergies or changes in existing ones
- Increased sensitivity to chemicals and medicine

Symptom checklist

The Canadian criteria (above), as you can see, are very thorough – again, much more so than the CDC classification. The following checklist, which I have devised, will help you to identify your own specific symptoms:

- Increased breathlessness with physical activity
- Change in body-temperature regulation (cold hands and feet)
- Concentration difficulties and confusion
- Word-retrieval problems (forgetting the right word)
- Dizziness, especially when standing up
- Increase in fatigue
- Digestive problems (such as indigestion, bloating, diarrhoea or constipation)
- Inability to tolerate either heat or cold
- Sweating
- Lengthy recovery period following exercise
- Change in weight (noticeable gain or loss)
- Poor memory
- Muscle pain and weakness
- Sudden sensitivities to food, drugs, and chemical substances
- Joint pain and headaches
- Decrease in mental and physical endurance
- Repeated flu-like symptoms

- Repeated sore throat
- Problems with sleep patterns
- Tender lymph glands

Fatigue and Post-exertional Malaise

Fatigue is a key feature of CFS, and while it may be intermittent and not a constant presence for all CFS sufferers, for many it is completely overwhelming. Yet fatigue is a contentious point in this disorder, in that many people with CFS are told either implicitly or explicitly to 'buck up and stop complaining'.

If you have CFS, you're not just tired in the normal sense, say, from staying up all night to finish a work report or because you've been rushing around, trying to tie up all the loose ends before you go on holiday. Your body is so overwhelmed by extreme exhaustion that with every movement you feel like you've run a marathon. And it's not as if a twenty-minute nap or a good night's sleep can refresh you – with CFS, nothing revives you. (I used to try to combat my fatigue with endless cups of coffee and tea, hoping for that pick-me-up boost. The result? I'd still be exhausted, but I'd also be wired – an odd combination of conflicting feelings, I assure you!)

The causes of fatigue

In the course of my research I have identified five main causes for fatigue in CFS. All of these point to biological factors, which is important given that many doctors and psychologists attribute fatigue exclusively to psychological causes (whether depression or fear of the pain and discomfort produced by reconditioning weak muscles).

1. Malfunctioning immune system

With an infection due to a virus, most people believe that the unpleasant symptoms – achiness, swollen glands, tiredness, chills and fever, etc. – are signs of the virus itself. However, these symptoms are, in fact, a sign that the immune system has kicked into action, has identified the infectious agent and is attacking it, diverting energy from other parts of the body to fight bugs. So while you may feel tired and dreadful during this process, it is all – even that runny, snotty nose – a good sign of immune function. Once the infection is defeated the activated immune system is switched off, you no longer feel the symptoms and you return to a healthy state.

With CFS, however, the body is unable to fight off infections effectively. The immune system is compromised and consequently you remain stuck, suspended in a state of ill health. So you experience all the discomfort of the immune system trying (but failing) to do its job – including fatigue – with none of the curative benefits.

2. Large intestine (or gut) blocked with bad bacteria

Although a controversial point in the literature (many doctors fail to see its relevance to the development of CFS[2], while others see it as central[3]) candida is often common among people with CFS and this is a major cause of fatigue. The gut is an important component of the immune system – as much as 80 per cent of immune-system cells rest in the large intestine – so if your intestines are overrun with bacterial overgrowth, your immune system could be compromised. As a result, you will not be processing your food properly and vital minerals and vitamins, essential for healthy and active living, will not reach your cells due to this blockage, which means you will feel extremely fatigued. I know people with CFS who eat the healthiest diets, but who could also be labelled as malnourished, simply because of the high levels of bacteria in their gut that prevent adequate nutrient absorption.

3. Poor circulation

Poor circulation is also a common symptom of CFS. Sufferers often complain of cold hands and feet because the tiny blood vessels which supply blood to these areas are failing to function normally. In fact, some people with CFS exhibit an ashen complexion because their blood supply is struggling to circulate to the skin.

This blood-flow impairment also plays a role in energy reduction. Your circulation brings nutrients to the cells and also aids in flushing away toxins and other waste materials. So it stands to reason that if your circulation is sluggish, your cells will have problems obtaining the vital nutrients they need to function.

4. Adrenal exhaustion

Adrenal exhaustion is another explanation for the fatigue linked to CFS.[4] The adrenal glands, which are located near the kidneys, produce hormones vital to life, and are part of a wider biological network known as the hypothalamic-pituitary-adrenal (HPA) axis (see also pp. 67–9), which is essential to governing healthy bodily functions such as heart rate, mood, body temperature, thirst and hunger. The adrenal glands are an important part of this system because they produce certain hormones in response to stress: adrenaline and cortisol. If you become overstressed, you might deplete your adrenals' ability to make these hormones, causing levels to drop and leading to a whole host of CFS symptoms, including fatigue. This is what is meant by adrenal exhaustion.

5. Mitochondrial dysfunction

Mitochondria[5] represent the cells' own personal fuel pump or furnace supply. The body cannot function correctly if its cells are not making enough energy. This is what we mean by mitochondrial dysfunction – and when this occurs, fatigue is a likely result.

Post-exertional malaise

While fatigue in patients with CFS is often global and disabling on its own, the pathological exhaustion can be worsened through either physical or cognitive exertion. Other symptoms exacerbated by this activity include increased general feelings of illness, reduction of mental function, increased muscle fatigue and soreness and a drop in endurance. Existing symptoms could also worsen. The symptoms of post-exertional malaise often appear immediately, but can also surface days or weeks following the activity.

According to Carruthers and van de Sande (2005)[6], such symptom decline points to abnormalities in immune-system regulation, toxicity due to oxidation and nitric oxide and low blood pressure.

There are also differences following exercise between CFS patients and their healthy counterparts in reaction to exertion, heart-rate efficiency, body temperature, cerebral oxygen, breathing, mental processing, recovery rates and oxygen transport to muscle and movement.

Six-month Rule

The six-month rule is also used as a diagnostic indicator and is applied to differentiate normal symptoms of, for example, a serious virus from which the body is merely taking a long time to recover, and a more prolonged disease state, like CFS. Although this is strictly applied by the CDC criteria, the Canadian criteria are in fact less stringent about the six-month rule, allowing some leeway in terms of time. In my view, the six-month rule should be largely ignored for the following reasons:

- The rule is completely arbitrary; it is not determined by medical factors and is not essential for a diagnosis. In other words, it is designed for diagnostic convenience. It's not as if, say for five months and thirty-odd days, you're just 'a little under the weather', but on the next day, with all the same symptoms, you suddenly have a serious illness.

- The lengthy wait means delay in essential diagnosis and treatment.

- The sooner you seek help, the better your outcome will be.

- Each person with CFS displays different symptoms and at different rates. In some cases symptoms come and go; in others things get slowly and progressively worse. In other words, CFS doesn't always play by a rigid six-month rule.

- In practical terms, the sooner you receive a diagnosis and get well, the sooner you can go back to work. You don't want to add unemployment and mortgage arrears to your list of worries.

So my message to you is this: don't hesitate. If you are worried about your symptoms, even if you've only been unwell for a month or two, I'd disregard the six-month rule and seek help now. In my view, if the onset of your symptoms can be traced to an infection, emotional or physical trauma, vaccination and you can rule out a history of other conditions – as far as possible – then CFS may well be the problem.

As I said earlier, you should *always* seek a diagnosis from your doctor first, but you will find that the better informed you are, the more likely it is that your examination will be thorough and that a CFS diagnosis can be unequivocally confirmed or ruled out. The remainder of this chapter is aimed at ensuring that you are equipped to achieve this.

When is CFS not CFS? Ruling out the medical mimickers

There is a saying in medicine, 'All that wheezes, ain't asthma', meaning that there are a number of diverse causes of breathing difficulties. And so it is with CFS, as a number of other medical conditions – some potentially serious – might be the source of your symptoms. Since CFS has a number of medical mimickers, in other words illnesses with similar symptoms, you should be aware of these to help with your own diagnosis.

In his book *Living with M.E.*,[7] Dr Charles Shepherd

provides a list of other possible causes of chronic fatigue symptoms which he has very kindly given me permission to reproduce here (if you suspect that you might be suffering from any of these, contact your doctor for more information):

Blood illnesses

- Anaemia
- Haemochromatosis

Side effects of certain prescription and over-the-counter medications

Gastro-intestinal illnesses

- Coeliac's disease
- Crohn's disease
- Food allergy/intolerance
- Irritable Bowel Syndrome (IBS)

Heart disorders

- Intermittent claudication
- Low blood pressure

Hormonal dysfunction

- Addison's disease
- Cushing's syndrome
- Pituitary tumours
- Hyperthyroidism
- Hypothyroidism

Infections

- Brucellosis
- Campylobacter
- Cytomegalovirus

- Giardia
- Hepatitis
- HIV
- Leptospirosis hardjo
- Lyme disease
- Mycoplasma
- Parvovirus B19
- Q fever
- Toxocara
- Toxoplasmosis
- Yersinia pseudotuberculosis

Liver disease
- Primary biliary cirrhosis
- Gilbert's disease

Malignancy
- Hodgkin's disease

Muscle disorders
- Myasthenia Gravis
- Polymyalgia rheumatica
- Polymyositis

Neurological disorders
- Multiple sclerosis
- Parkinson's disease

Poisoning
- Carbon monoxide
- Lead

Psychiatric disorders
- Anxiety

- Depression
- Hyperventilation syndrome
- Post-traumatic stress disorder
- Seasonal affective disorder (SAD)
- Somatisation
- Stress and overwork

Respiratory disorders
- Sarcoidosis
- Tuberculosis

Rheumatic disorders
- Sjögren's syndrome
- Systemic lupus erythematosus

Other conditions
- Alcohol abuse
- Raised blood calcium
- Osteomalacia
- Sick building syndrome
- Sleep apnoea and narcolepsies
- Sexual dysfunction

Overlapping disorders
- Athletic overtraining
- Ciguatera poisoning
- Fibromyalgia
- Fluid-retention syndrome
- Gulf War syndrome
- Organophosphate poisoning
- Post-polio syndrome

I'd also add to the list, arthritis, bipolar disorder, anorexia and bulimia, viral and bacterial infections and obesity. There are so many illnesses, syndromes and disorders that mimic CFS, it is essential that you get the most thorough and reliable diagnosis. If you do have problems with your doctor who might not believe in CFS or, for whatever reason, thinks you do not have it, you should study this list with great care in order to rule out possible mimickers.

Your Own Vital Role in Your Diagnosis

Although hopefully your doctor will be amenable to offering you a thorough investigation in order to reach a diagnosis, you also have a vital part to play in the process.

Your medical history

Because diagnosing CFS is rife with problems, a good place for you to start is to take a few moments to analyse the course of your symptoms and your overall medical history. Look at the following categories – the more clear you are in your own mind about these, the more expedient the diagnostic process will be:

- **Your symptoms** Was the onset gradual or sudden? What are the triggers? Consider the variation of symptoms throughout the day, which you experience and when and which seem to get better and worse.

- **Your history of other illnesses** What 'mimickers' of CFS (see box, p. 29) have you personally experienced and can bring to the attention of your doctor?

- **Previous treatments** Write these down so you can discuss with your doctor what has worked and what hasn't.

- **Your mental-health history** As I have already said (see p. 14), I don't think depression causes CFS, but the two can, and often do, co-exist. So it is important to consider this issue.

- **Recent travels** Have you recently travelled abroad? If so, did you have any vaccinations? What were the standards of hygiene like where you were? Was the water safe to drink? Was the food cooked properly?
- **Your sexual history** Did you have unprotected sex with others whose own history you were unsure of before the onset of your symptoms?
- **Your lifestyle** Have you undergone a lengthy period of stress? Do you burn the candle at both ends? Have you recently experienced a bereavement, job loss, pregnancy or some other major life change?
- **Genetic history** Has someone else in your family been diagnosed with CFS or struggled to recover following a severe viral or bacterial infection? People with CFS have shown genetic differences compared with their healthy counterparts, so if someone in your family has been diagnosed with CFS or is exhibiting fatigue and other CFS symptoms, you might be more vulnerable.
- **Allergies and sensitivities to chemicals** Food allergies and chemical sensitivities are not unknown in people with CFS and these reactions can make you feel exhausted, achy and bring you out in rashes. Also, if you live near a farm, organophosphate poisoning might also be a culprit.

Sleep Pattern Record

Since so many people with CFS report problems with sleep, I would also like you to keep a sleep diary. Once you have begun to recover and your body clock starts to correct itself, you should see an improvement in your ability to sleep. However, until this point, it will be helpful to chart your current nightly sleep patterns. Please record your symptoms for a week or two. This will establish a 'base rate' or starting point from which you can gauge improvement.

Use the following template to help you with this goal.

	Monday	Tuesday	Wednesday	Thursday	Friday	Saturday	Sunday
Midnight– 2 a.m.							
2–4 a.m.							
4–6 a.m.							
6–8 a.m.							
8–10 a.m.							
10–12 noon							
12–2 p.m.							
2–4 p.m.							
4–6 p.m.							
6–8 p.m.							
8–10 p.m.							
10 p.m – midnight							

Current Activity Levels

Using the above template again (I would suggest either photo-copying it or recording it in your own writing in a notebook), I now want you to analyse your current abilities. Take an average day from when you were healthy, prior to the onset of your symptoms and record your typical activities: you can simply enter 'watched TV', 'made breakfast', 'had a nap', 'slept', etc. Don't worry if for much of the night, you simply write asleep. It's important to document all your activities and behaviours.

Once you've recorded your 'healthy' day, I want you to repeat the exercise, but this time write down what a typical twenty-four-hour period is like with CFS.

Seeing the differences between what you were able to do before you became ill and now might be a bit of a shock, when confronted in black and white, but it is important for a good, firm diagnosis. It's also important for you and your recovery. I want you to be fully aware of how this debilitating illness affects your life, specifically – because every case is individual. The important thing is to be as accurate as possible about your abilities. Don't push yourself further or harder because you are writing the activities down. Just be honest.

Share all this information with your doctor, even if he or she merely gives it a quick glance. At the very least, you will be keeping them 'in the loop'. I would also recommend that you use this diary method to chart your progress and track your rate of recovery. As your body begins – and continues – to heal, your ability to sleep should improve.

Top Tips to Help You Communicate with Your Doctor

Visiting the doctor can be intimidating at the best of times, but the encounter can be even more fraught when you're in the throes of CFS. You are no doubt feeling exhausted, vulnerable, and might even have particular communication difficulties, such as concentration and memory impairments or word displacements (problems with word retrieval or identification). Here are some tips to help you with the communication process:

- **Bring a friend or family member** This person can provide moral support and also help to communicate your main concerns and needs. Make sure your companion is well versed in your situation so that they can better act as your advocate.

- **Draw up a list of your main concerns** Some doctors will give you as much time as you need, while others are pressed for time and will all but shuffle you out of the door, before you've even sat down. The better prepared you are for the consultation, the more you will get out of it.

- **Be polite but firm** You have a serious illness and you deserve respect. Don't be fobbed off with a dismissive attitude or inadequate treatment. Doctors are there to help you.

And finally, always make sure you obtain full diagnosis of CFS from your doctor – the above guidelines should help you enormously in reaching this goal.

CHAPTER THREE

Fibromyalgia and Depression: Close Cousins of CFS

I've decided to write separately about fibromyalgia (FM or FMS) and depression as there is often confusion about their roles in relation to CFS, with endless debates between doctors, psychologists and others as to the distinctions between them. Some claim that they are all different names for the same affliction, while others believe that they are separate conditions, albeit with a certain degree of overlap – all of which makes diagnosis and treatment even more problematic, so clarification is essential for you. In my view, all three are distinct, separate illnesses. My main concern is that people with CFS or fibromyalgia are often dismissed as having depression when, in fact, they do not.

Fibromyalgia (FM or FMS)

Millions of people around the world are thought to have FMS (fibromyalgia syndrome).[1] Like CFS, it is a chronic, disabling illness. However, unlike in CFS, the chief symptom here is extreme pain in the muscles and tendons. So although fatigue is often an associated symptom, people with fibromyalgia would describe first and foremost the extreme muscle pain they experience. Also, the pain does not appear to be 'fixed', often moving around from place to place in the body.

Unfortunately, as with CFS, a lot of medical professionals still lump fibromyalgia into the 'hypochondriac's charter', but the illness is very real. The exact cause is still open to debate, but it is thought that chronic stress, a virus or some kind of trauma (such as a car crash or sexual or physical abuse), or a combination, causes hormones and other body chemistry to go haywire and malfunction.[2] Researchers are still unclear as to why this is the case, but in Chapter Five I spell out my theory as to how two such different causes – the psychological and the physical – can lead to one illness.

Here are some of the many symptoms associated with the disorder. How many of them do you have?

- Painful muscles and tendons
- Flu-like achiness and discomfort
- General body aches and pains
- Sleep disturbances
- Worsening of symptoms following exercise
- Concentration difficulties and confusion
- Ongoing back pain
- Stiff muscles
- Anxiety symptoms
- Depression
- Anger
- Extreme exhaustion

If you think you might have FMS, you should contact your doctor. To find out more about the condition, see Resources, p. 193.

Depression

Anyone with CFS who has sought medical help will no doubt have been told at some point that their symptoms are caused by depression. But is there any truth to this statement? Well, yes . . . and . . . no.

As a clinical psychologist who has treated many people with mood disorders and written on the subject, I can absolutely 100 per cent assure you that CFS and depression are two completely distinct illnesses. However, they share some common traits and there can be some symptom overlap. You could, of course, be suffering from depressive symptoms independently of CFS, due, most likely to a genetic vulnerability to developing this low mood condition. Or you could also develop these psychological symptoms as a result of the reduced quality of life associated with the ongoing nature of a serious chronic illness. Or you could experience low mood due to biological disturbances caused by CFS itself. Viruses, dysfunctional brain chemicals and cytokines (immune-system chemicals triggered to fight infectious agents) all lead to depressive symptoms. However, it is not a given that just because you have CFS, you also automatically have depression.

If you suffer with CFS, you don't just experience physical pain; your entire life can be hijacked, leading to a whole host of seemingly insurmountable worries and anxieties, social isolation and loneliness, relationship breakdown and financial woes. Even the struggle to perform day-to-day personal hygiene tasks can be enough to cause pathological despondency. If you are unlucky enough to have an unsympathetic doctor or psychologist who latches on to any symptom of depression you express as a sign of mental disease and refuses to entertain the notion of physical causation, then this section is particularly important for you.

The Diagnostic Criteria: Differences Between Depression and CFS

Here are some of the main differences between the two illnesses:

- While both patient groups complain of fatigue, with CFS the exhaustion is much more constant, global and disabling. It is the cardinal symptom of CFS and tends to be exacerbated by exercise (post-exertional malaise). In fact, I would say post-exertional malaise could be a good diagnostic indicator for CFS, as it is not associated with mood disorder.

- The existence of particular physical symptoms, or 'flu-like' symptoms, such as swollen, tender glands, sore throat, cough, temperature dysfunction and twitching muscles are hallmarks of CFS, but not of depression.

- With depression, people often feel apathetic and lose all interest in or gain little pleasure from activities they previously enjoyed (anhedonia). Most CFS people can't wait to recover, so they can again actively participate in their life's previous joys. As a result, they often feel frustrated by and impatient with their lack of recovery.

- Depressed people often *don't want* to get out of bed in the morning because they believe the day will lead to nothing other than hopelessness and despair. In contrast, people with CFS *can't* get out of bed because they simply don't have the energy or strength to do so.

- When people with CFS go out or exert themselves a little too much, they can feel both mentally and physically worse, often leading to a lengthy setback. However, when individuals with depression push themselves and, say, go to a party, they often feel better for having made the effort.

- Mental exertion in CFS can lead to a worsening of physical and psychological symptoms. In depression, there is no detrimental effect.

- There is evidence of immune malfunction (symptoms) in people with CFS (such as swollen glands, fatigue, increased temperature), where there is not with depression.

- In people with depression, there is decreased self-esteem, whereas in CFS, self-esteem is intact.

- With depression, suicidal thoughts can be pervasive. In CFS, they tend to be temporary.

CFS and depression are both serious illnesses, both of which have often been dismissed as malingering by the medical and psychological professions and both of which can lead to suicide, so it is vital that you monitor your mood levels as well as your physical symptoms.

Are you depressed?

If you have CFS, you are naturally and normally going to feel depressed and anxious to some degree at some points along the way. In fact, *not* to have a strong emotional reaction to a devastating illness strikes me as abnormal and could even point to denial. In Chapter Eight, I will help you to deal with these emotions, but for now, just let yourself be human. Allow yourself to feel what you feel, but if your emotions become unbearable or hard to cope with, you must, absolutely *must*, seek immediate help from your doctor. CFS is hard enough to deal with on its own, without adding other strains to the pot.

However, because symptoms of depression, including concentration difficulties, confusion, fatigue, weepiness, anxiety, sleep disturbances, are also evident in CFS, it might sometimes be complicated to differentiate easily between the two syndromes.

If you suspect you might be depressed, answer the following questions[3] covering the standard diagnostic themes your doctor will be looking for:

1. Do you feel a profound sense of sadness, hopelessness or despair?
2. Have you lost interest in the activities that normally give you pleasure?
3. Have you noticed a significant change in your appetite, either eating less or more?
4. Have you developed problems or changes in sleeping patterns, either sleeping too much or too little?
5. Do you feel lethargic and apathetic?

6. Do you feel more tired than usual?
7. Are you experiencing a persistent sense of hopelessness or guilt?
8. Are you suffering from problems in your ability to think or concentrate?
9. Are you contemplating suicide?

If you answer 'Yes' to five or more of these questions and have been experiencing the changes for at least two weeks, you could be suffering some degree of depression and you must seek help now. However, if you do not satisfy these criteria, your symptoms are not caused by a depressive illness. If your doctor tries to dismiss your symptoms with a depressive label, point his or her attention to this diagnostic checklist.

Three types of depression

If you have CFS and you also suffer from depression, it is essential that you clarify the exact nature of your mood disorder. One of the biggest problems with the standard diagnostic depression checklist above is that while it captures all the main symptom categories of depression, it fails to identify the underlying cause. So you might be depressed; you just won't know exactly why. And it follows that if doctors cannot figure out the cause of your depression, your treatment might be unsuitable. Also, just like with CFS, there is currently no definitive diagnostic test for depression and diagnosis is generally made on the basis of subjective self-report.

While many doctors and psychologists lump all cases of depression together in the one category, my research has shown that there are at least three distinct types and that these must be treated by different means. Antidepressants and talk therapies are not interchangeable; in fact, indiscriminate and inappropriate use of either could lead to no relief or even worsening of symptoms. So to maximise treatment success, it is always best to match the therapy to the precise type of depression. These, in my clinical view, are the three main distinctive categories of depression:

1. Primary (or biological) depression

With this type of mood disorder, certain brain chemicals (neuro-transmitters) malfunction leaving you with a pathologically low mood and those other symptoms of depression. In such cases, talk therapies on their own are unlikely to treat the problem effectively and antidepressants probably work best. So if your symptoms of depression came on 'out of the blue' and cannot strongly be linked to a stressful life event and if antidepressants work so well that you no longer feel the need to talk to a therapist, biological depression is the likely cause.

Some people feel uncomfortable about taking antidepressants because they erroneously believe them to be the 'weak' option, but biological depression is as valid a medical illness as diabetes or cancer. I would say, however, that if you have CFS in addition to depression, you might feel your system becomes overwhelmed with strong medication and, as a result, has problems coping with the drugs. If so, talk to your doctor about starting off with a smaller dose of antidepressants and then building up as required.

2. Secondary depression (a common side effect of medication or a symptom of underlying physical illness)

This is the most often overlooked category of depressive illness and, I believe, the source of much confusion around the disorder, leading to a delay in diagnosis and effective treatment.

Certain medical illnesses or, indeed over-the-counter and prescription medications[4] can actually produce depressive symptoms, even when there is no evidence of psychological distress or personal difficulty. In other words, physical illnesses can also produce psychological symptoms even when there is no emotional crisis whatsoever. Emotional distress can also be symptomatic of unpleasant side effects of certain medications, alcohol or illegal drugs. (See Appendix A, p. 185, for a complete list of depression mimickers.)

3. Tertiary depression

Sometimes referred to as exogenous or reactive depression, this refers to an adverse emotional reaction to a major stressful life event, such as divorce, job loss, bereavement or illness. In these cases, people can usually identify the likely cause of their symptoms and feel psychologically traumatised by the stressor. Any major (or sometimes even minor) personal calamity can leave us shaken to the core and knock us off our perch of mental well-being.

So if there is a definite trigger – and CFS *is* a definite potential trigger – you should consider tertiary depression a possibility. Hopefully, your doctor will be able to refer you to a psychologist or counsellor for talk therapy.

In a nutshell . . .

- Depression and CFS are two distinct illnesses, although there can be overlap in symptoms, leading to confusion in diagnosis.
- There are no definitive diagnostic tests for either depression or CFS, again, potentially leading to confusion in diagnosis.
- People with CFS can also develop depression as a separate disorder.
- Likewise, people with depression can also come down with CFS as a separate condition.
- People with CFS can develop symptoms of depression as a feature of the neurochemical breakdown that can occur with the illness.
- People with CFS can develop depression due to the confines of long-term illness and reduced quality of life.

Now, with your diagnosis of CFS hopefully confirmed, we can turn to the causes of the condition.

CHAPTER FOUR

Mainstream Theories about the Causes of CFS

As we've just seen, even the very basics of CFS – such as diagnosing the disorder – are rife with conflict, confusion and debate. This contention reflects the long battle to legitimise CFS as a valid health problem and although doctors are now just beginning to take the whole area seriously, the struggle continues. To be sure, we have made great strides in understanding CFS, but there is still a long way to go, and the dispute over the causes of the illness remains one of the biggest obstacles to its effective treatment within mainstream medicine. Opinion falls into two distinct camps: the psychological and the biological. Proponents of the psychological view dominate the field, and theirs is a powerful position, leaving little room for alternative explanations.

The History of CFS Treatments

It should seem obvious that psychological treatments alone cannot cure medical problems, although they can help support people in the process of recovery, because that's what they are designed to do. So many people ask me to explain the reasons why psychological treatments have come to dominate the field, given this inconsistency. The following brief history of CFS should help to make the situation clearer.

Many people believe that CFS is a modern disease, so it might surprise you to learn that telltale symptoms of the disorder were identified hundreds of years ago. Back then, there was no recognised medical syndrome to account for the odd cluster of unusual symptoms that we now call CFS, but they were thought to be physical in origin.

The disorder first became formalised in 1750, when Sir Richard Manningham, a physician, labelled it as febricula (little fever). Over one hundred years later, the now familiar collection of CFS-like traits – particularly exhaustion, high temperature and malaise – obtained a new label of neurasthenia. It wasn't until 1930 that the medical establishment first used the more familiar modern name of myalgic encephalomyelitis (ME), and although the term CFS (coined in the 1980s) is often now preferred, ME is still commonly used today.

So far, so physical. But in 1955, despite the long-term, historical acceptance of 'flu-like' and, therefore, physical symptoms, the outbreak of a mysterious, seemingly viral illness at a London hospital, prompted the current medical view that CFS symptoms are the result of nothing more than patient hysteria. Here's what happened:

In the summer of 1955, several patients were admitted to the Royal Free Hospital with a range of suspected infectious symptoms, including gastric problems, respiratory complaints, sore throat, increased temperature and swollen glands – the typical hallmarks of a nasty viral or bacterial bug. Instead of making the expected recovery, however, many of these patients developed a new collection of puzzling symptoms, including brain dysfunction, severe muscle aches, exhaustion, malaise, cold extremities and visual disturbances. In addition, some of the staff who had been treating these patients subsequently became ill themselves. The Royal Free doctors were initially united in their diagnosis that the cause of symptoms was some form of viral or bacterial infection agent. However, they were unable to find the precise source of the infection.

Even given the limited methods of investigation at the time, it is likely that further medical research enquiries would have been undertaken along the infectious line of enquiry, had it not been for two psychiatrists – Dr Colin McEvedy and Dr Alfred William

Beard – who concluded (albeit some years later) that the symptoms of the Royal Free outbreak had not been physical at all, but that they were the product of mass ward hysteria.[1] According to them (based on second-hand evidence viewed fifteen years later), a patient at the hospital had become overly anxious and hysterical (although the exact reason for this remains unexplored), triggering a neurotic chain reaction throughout the ward and, indeed, among some staff members. So, not so much a viral infection, but a psychological one, they argued.

Although by this time the medical community had pretty much lost interest in the Royal Free disease, the psychiatric label took hold and stuck. The psychiatrists had completely ignored the physical signs of illness – the swollen glands, sore throat, confusion, breathing difficulties, etc. – but the damage was done, and from then on, anyone with CFS symptoms was branded neurotic, malingering and mentally unstable.

Drs McEvedy and Beard wrote about the Royal Free. The paper was so influential that CFS became a fully-fledged psychosomatic illness. And, even though changes were made in 2009, reclassifying CFS from a psychiatric condition to a medical one, old habits die hard and the hysteria view is still influential.

While psychological traits are common in CFS, whether because they are a symptom of the problem or due to the misery of reduced circumstances, the point is that currently psychologists and doctors fail to grasp the exact nature of this emotional distress, and the psychosomatic view of CFS remains, the result being that far from being helped, many patients are insulted, dismissed and, ultimately, abandoned.

From the darkness comes light, however. A few pioneering people – myself included – have recognised the scientific flaws and limitations of these long-held diagnosis and treatment viewpoints and have worked tirelessly to discover the true nature of the disorder and to devise effective treatments. We are, however, a lonely breed, and we are fighting a very powerful lobby.

I will discuss the biological and psychological causes of CFS in the next chapter. However, since current accepted treatments are based on psychological understandings of the illness, as we have already seen, it is important that you are fully aware of these practices, as they underpin the treatments that are available. The main treatments offered come in the form of cognitive behavioural therapy and graded exercise therapy.

Cognitive Behavioural Therapy (CBT)

Many of you will probably already have had experiences of CBT. The therapy is currently the most influential form of psychotherapy around the world, not just for CFS. Initially devised in the 1950s as cognitive therapy, its original purpose was to treat depression, but now the treatment has been adapted and is used to help patients cope with all kinds of psychological and medical problems, including eating disorders, substance misuse, anxiety and phobias. Unlike the other major psychotherapeutic traditions, which are dominated by the therapist, CBT was hailed as a breakthrough because it teaches patients and clients the skills to cope with their own difficulties. In essence, therefore, with CBT, the patient becomes his or her own therapist. In many ways, this can be empowering for the individual when, of course, the strategy is used appropriately. However, often with CFS it is not. As a result, patients often fail to improve and are also usually blamed for their lack of recovery. Later (see Chapter Eight), I will explain when and how CBT can be effective with this condition.

The core philosophy of CBT is that your thoughts, emotions and behaviour are so tightly interwoven that they all influence one another. So, if you *feel* a certain way, you will develop corresponding thoughts and behaviours that are compatible with these emotions. As an example, if you feel depressed, your thoughts and actions will reflect your low mood – you will become bleak and negative in outlook, apathetic and will often isolate yourself as a result. In contrast, when you are happy, you feel joyful and manifest your elation in your thoughts and behaviours: you focus only on the positive and on all that's right with the world, you greet your fellow humans with a hearty smile and enthuse about the joys of being alive.

CBT also addresses the subjective nature of human beings. This means that we are generally unable to analyse events in our lives from an objective standpoint, being too emotionally charged to think clearly. So when faced with a crisis, for example, we find it difficult to step back and maintain a detached, calm view of events and come up with a constructive response. Instead, we often panic, become anxious and automatically resort to 'worst-case-scenario' thinking, which, in turn, makes us feel worse and can place us on the path for making the wrong decisions. CBT helps to develop a more balanced approach to analysing life's stressors, so that we don't immediately resort to panic.

CBT in action

The following is a light-hearted illustration of human nature according to the CBT paradigm.

Three men have been out of work for an extended period of time and have an interview lined up for a new position they are desperate to secure. As each man leaves his house on the morning of the interview, suddenly, and without warning, there is a roar of thunder, the skies open and rain starts pelting down. Since the weather forecast had predicted nothing but sunny skies for the day and this downpour was completely unexpected, all three men had left their umbrellas at home and were, consequently, soaked to the skin. How does each one respond?

The first man became very negative and pessimistic. The very embodiment of doom and gloom: 'I just knew this would happen! Nothing ever goes right for me! Every time I make positive changes in my life and try to get ahead, it all just gets thrown back in my face. There's no point in going to the interview now. What's the point? I'm such a loser. They'd all see this and just laugh at me.' With this downcast, bleak demeanour, man number one went straight home and never made it to the interview.

The second man fared little better, but his response was completely different. He was so upset by his dishevelled, waterlogged appearance that he began to panic about the interview. What would they think? Then, anxious and distressed, he started to sweat, his heart began to race and he felt weak at the knees. His pulse was racing so fast, he thought his heart was going to burst through his chest. The symptoms were so severe that he ditched the interview entirely and rushed to the nearest accident and emergency facility, terrified and convinced he was having a heart attack.

The third man reacted with optimism. He was happy it was just rain. The situation could have been worse, he thought – it could have been a flock of pigeons! He skipped off happily to the interview and got the job.

One situation, three men, three responses: this is the essence of CBT.

In later chapters, we will look at the many CBT strategies that are effective in treating CFS. When it is appropriately applied, this therapy is actually very successful.

Graded Exercise Therapy (GET)

Graded Exercise Therapy or GET often goes hand in hand with CBT as the main therapy offered to people with CFS. The strategy is rehabilitative in focus. Its purpose is to help people regain stamina and fitness following a serious illness, through a series of stepped exercises which build on previous successes. So, for example, in week one you'd walk a quarter of a block, week two, half a block and so on. In theory GET is very successful, but only when the body is in a state in which recovery is possible – i.e. when a person has already overcome their illness and is now well on the way to full health. Unfortunately, the problem with CFS is that people who are still in the grips of illness are physically unable to participate in such a gruelling programme. In fact, GET can often make people with CFS worse.[2]

CBT and GET: How *Not* to Apply Them

Here's a scenario to help you understand your symptoms better, and the reasons why your current treatments and healthcare professionals have let you down.

Let's say, for example, you broke your leg, after a fall. However, instead of obtaining an initial examination, an X-ray and perhaps undergoing an operation to reset the bone, when you pitch up at the emergency room, you are informed that there is nothing medically wrong and you are sent away, without any tests or investigations whatsoever.

You go home and the pain in your leg fails to improve. So you return to your doctor, who insists that everything is normal and to be expected. After all, you did have a fall, so you should expect a certain degree of achiness, swelling and limited movement. You are sent away again. However, the pains in your leg still fail to improve and, again, you return to your doctor. By this time, you are becoming increasingly anxious, but no one seems to take you seriously. You don't require a doctor, you are told – you need a psychologist. And, although you still believe your symptoms are physical, you dutifully, show up at the appointed time with the therapist. The psychologist agrees with the doctor and a course of CBT is advised to help restore your emotional balance and a graded exercise programme (GET) is drawn up to strengthen your leg muscles which have now wasted. You are instructed to walk a little further each day until your withered limb regains its conditioning and full fitness. Then, and only then, will your anxiety levels reduce. Dutifully, you leave the office and do your best to follow the psychologist's carefully laid-out plan. Except, of course, you cannot. You try to push yourself, despite the pain, but the next day, your leg is worse still. You get no better. Your doctor and psychologist eventually tire of your apparent mental blocks to recovery. You give up. They give up. You are then left alone with your symptoms.

Of course, in the case of the broken-leg scenario, the doctors' response is clearly absurd, even ludicrous. However, replace the broken leg with CFS and this is precisely what happens to countless sufferers.

In Conclusion

Although many doctors and psychologists argue in support of using CBT and GET for CFS,[3] alluding to very high success rates, their information may be flawed in that it fails to take into account some important considerations. For example, most people who participate in CBT and GET treatment studies tend to be only moderately or mildly affected by the disorder and, therefore, well enough to access treatment and to participate in the research. Those who experience the most severe form of the illness – myself included – would be too debilitated to take part in the first place. Also, many patients feel pressure to provide 'good' scores, either to be polite to someone they know, as is the social expectation, or for fear of having treatment and care denied them in future if they fail to respond favourably. A study conducted at Stony Brook University, New York, in 2009 points to this problem of 'socially desirable answers', whereby patients reported feeling much better than they actually were out of a sense of duty to their practitioners.[4]

So while both CBT and GET do have a significant place in the care of people with CFS, they should only be used once the underlying causes of the condition have been addressed and are being treated and recovery is under way. We need to look at the whole picture and take things one step at a time, beginning with the causes of CFS, which is where we are going next.

CHAPTER FIVE
Explaining the True Causes of CFS

It should be obvious by now that the psychosomatic theories about the causes of CFS espoused by many doctors and psychologists are not only erroneous and patronising, but that they also fail to acknowledge or explain the huge raft or biological symptoms (as specified in the Canadian criteria) and that they ignore the evidence from leading pioneers in research of the illness, such as Byron Hyde from the Nightingale Foundation, Jay Goldstein, Jacob Teitelbaum and Kenny De Meirleir, among others.

My theory aims to explain the illness more fully. In my view, the following factors are all involved in the development of CFS:

- There is usually a genetic susceptibility.
- There needs to be a biological or psychological trigger.
- The body has to malfunction in response to that trigger or 'short circuit'.
- The body must be unable to recover and regain health.
- The stress caused by protracted and debilitating symptoms then serve to reinforce the illness.

As a result of all this, the body stays suspended in a state of biological and psychological 'chaos'. In other words, CFS is caused when the body's innate healing systems short-circuit and fail to correct themselves. Although viral and bacterial infections are seen as the main triggers of the illness in genetically susceptible people,[1] there are also other biological triggers that have been noted in the literature[2] (vaccinations, and environmental poisons for example). Psychological trauma in the form of bereavement or divorce or physical trauma, such as car accidents, surgery or childbirth also produce symptoms of CFS.

In both cases, whether psychological or physical, the stressful factor produces the same physiological reactions. When the body is under threat, it responds by activating certain nervous, immunological and endocrinal chemicals (such as adrenaline, cortisol and platelet-activating factor) to help it cope. In healthy people, these biochemicals soon settle back down to normal and they go about their business as normal. With CFS, however, the body fails to settle back down in a predicted manner, leaving the person in a state of ill health from which it is difficult or near impossible to recover.

In some cases it will be a one-off trauma that triggers this meltdown, while in others the body becomes weakened following a lengthy period of stress, rendering it more susceptible to breakdown, brought on by an infection. Furthermore, because chronic illness breeds more stress and distress, the body becomes locked into an ever-more weakened state, leading to the development of CFS.

Diversity of Symptoms

The enormous diversity of symptoms in CFS means that it is not a one-size-fits-all illness, which is why it is often so difficult to diagnose and research. The following illustration may help you to understand this aspect of the condition better.

When I describe the breakdown of the body's normal functioning in CFS, I often use the analogy of a line of Christmas tree lights. So for example, if we have one hundred bulbs on a tree, it will only be fully illuminated if they all work; and in the same way, the human body needs all its different physiological and psychological sub-systems to function in harmony. If any number of bulbs is not working, the tree cannot be lit up completely. So on one tree it might be bulbs ten, twenty-one or thirty-five in the sequence that are faulty, on another, it might be only the first one, while on a third it could be the final ten bulbs – but whichever bulb is missing, the end result is still the same: an unlit Christmas tree. And similarly, no two people with CFS will display exactly the same pattern of symptoms of biological breakdown.

Because the body is governed by a highly complex network of gland controls, the potential for breakdown is limitless. So for some CFS patients, a virus might be the culprit, burning out certain aspects of the immune system. For others, prolonged stress might have led to the malfunction of the adrenal glands. Or it might be a combination of both these scenarios, or it could be a car accident that leads to a breakdown of the body clock. Furthermore, the various sub-systems of each gland centre are also themselves multi-faceted leading to further unique variations of bodily breakdown in patients.

The Body Breakdown

Let's now take a look at the main factors leading up to CFS, including the role of predisposing, triggering and perpetuating factors, specifically the influence of stress, genetic traits, viral and bacterial infections, vaccinations, environmental poisons and emotional or physical trauma. We will also look at the specific biological mechanisms that become faulty as a result of this physical and psychological onslaught on the body. They include hypothalamic-pituitary-adrenal axis, the autonomic nervous system, the immune system, cell mitochondria and gastro-intestinal breakdown.

Here's a visual model of my theory:

Predisposing factors

Genetic predisposition

Nervous, immunological and hormonal systems

Reduced stress tolerance

Gender

Vulnerability to potential illness

+

Personal history of stress

Psychological stress　　　Physical stress　　　No discernible stress

Triggering factors

Infections　　　Vaccinations　　　Environmental poisons and allergens　　　Psychological and physical trauma

Body breakdown

Autonomic nervous system (ANS)
Hypothalamic–pituitary–adrenal (HPA) axis
Limbic system
Immune system
Gastro-intestinal system

CFS symptoms

Maintaining factors

Stress (e.g. job loss, financial pressures, loss of independence relationship breakdown, emotional distress)

CFS symptoms

Predisposing Factors

Genetic predisposition

CFS experts have pointed to a likely genetic predisposition to developing CFS.[3] This is not surprising. Our genes govern most areas of our lives. They are the building blocks of life and consist mainly of proteins, called amino acids. They are responsible for the functioning of all living organisms and determine pretty much everything about us – hair colour, height, weight, shape – that is most obvious to the naked eye. Internally, our genes also control our reactions to stress, hormone production, brain chemistry and the propensity to develop certain diseases, like CFS.

The role of stress

The role of stress is pivotal in CFS at all the different stages of the illness: predisposing, triggering and perpetuating, although the extent to which stress is reported varies.[4] A minority of people claim no stress at all prior to the onset of symptoms. In my view, this is often because people equate stress with emotional difficulties and tend to ignore the physical strain that can occur, such as extreme temperatures and physical endurance, pushing themselves too hard at work and ignoring signs of health decline because of responsibilities. Furthermore, the general consensus is that stress in the main produces and perpetuates CFS.[5] Some people, however, are just genetically more prone to feeling overburdened by life's pressures, due to their biological make-up and so are said to be predisposed to unhealthy reactions to life's strains. When doctors talk of a physical ability to cope with stress, they often refer to something called the allostatic load (or AL). Everyone has a different AL capacity: some people are able to take years of hard knocks before burnout eventually occurs, while others find that their bodies conk out under far less pressure. So the extent to which people can cope with stress varies enormously. However, people with CFS are thought to have a malfunctioning AL mechanism, rendering them more vulnerable than most to stress. So while our AL is down to a genetic lottery, its interaction with stressful triggers, either physical or emotional, can lead us one step closer to CFS.

We are only human. The constant demands and pressures of modern life seem not only limitless, but serve also as a toxic barrier to good emotional and physical wellbeing. We have only twenty-four hours in the day in which to look after children, commute to work, please the boss, juggle domestic duties, walk the dog, shop for food (just compiling this list alone is exhausting!). And all of these are potential triggering factors – as are viruses, surgical procedures, childbirth, divorce, bereavement or any serious strain. It is not always possible to cope with the slings and arrows of outrageous fortune, to quote Shakespeare, but we push ourselves anyway. And, sooner or later, something has to give. Usually, it is our health.

As a result of life's demands, we live on adrenaline to an unhealthy degree and respond to the pressures we so often misconceive as normal by giving up sleep, relying on caffeine, junk food, alcohol, drugs – anything to give us that vital energy boost. To keep going, to keep up, we push ourselves even when our bodies have given out, but fail to take the much needed time to replenish our internal resources and depleted energy stores. Since women still tend to perform most of the domestic duties and often hold down a full-time job as well, it is perhaps not surprising that females tend to be over-represented in the CFS patient statistics. Perhaps the condition should be renamed toxic-life syndrome.

The final straw for many does eventually come and the body implodes. It just cannot take the strain any more. The fuse is blown and our gland master centres which govern our health descend into chaos from which our body fails to recover or recover effectively. So when it experiences a stressful event, the body responds internally by releasing an avalanche of chemicals, such as adrenaline and cortisol, in reaction. In normal, healthy people, these chemicals eventually settle down and regular function is resumed. With CFS, however, it is likely instead that the body is unable to right itself and remains in a dysfunctional pattern of chemical chaos. Of course, when these processes work normally, we don't tend to feel any symptoms at all. It is only when problems arise that we begin to feel the debilitating signs of ill health.

Stress leaves us vulnerable to getting CFS in the first place, but it also plays a reinforcing role and perpetuates the symptoms. Chronic illness is, in itself, stressful, especially with a condition like CFS in which symptoms are so globally disabling; every body system is affected and every sense seems to be under assault. Then there is also loss of income and career, relationships suffer and friends disappear. Children have to cope with a disabled parent. And doctors don't seem to be able to help. All these stresses conspire and feed back into an already struggling body, causing more pressure, more strain, more internal weakness and more damage. The cycle of ill health continues.

Triggering Factors

On its own, a genetic predisposition to develop CFS would probably be insufficient to cause the condition. It is more likely that a particular trigger or series of traumatic events would be needed to result ultimately in the development of CFS. So while your genes might set you up, it is the triggers that give you the final push.

There is an infinite number of potential triggers, so I have limited discussion here to the main ones identified in the medical literature. They include viral and bacterial infections, vaccinations, environmental poisons and allergens and psychological and physical trauma.

Infections

Viral infections are considered the major trigger of CFS.[6] Even healthcare professionals who dismiss the idea that the illness is biological, still acknowledge the role of viruses as precipitator.[7] The following are some of the more commonly identified viruses in CFS:

Epstein-Barr virus (EBV)

Probably the most widely known suspect in CFS is the Epstein-Barr virus (EBV). This virus is a member of the herpes family, which is the responsible agent for infectious mononucleosis or 'mono', as it is commonly referred to in the USA or glandular fever as it is called in the United Kingdom. Sometimes referred to as the 'kissing disease' (because it is transmitted through saliva and is highly evident in adolescents), the EBV is so prevalent in the adult population that around 90 per cent of people have been exposed to it by the time they reach thirty.[8] The vast majority of people seem to be immune to the bug and, therefore, will show few, if any, symptoms at all. For others, however, symptoms can range from pretty mild to severe, leaving people fatigued and suffering from enlarged glands and sore throats, lasting up to three months in normal cases. Once symptoms have subsided, the virus stays in the body for life, and while in most cases this is not problematic, the EBV can reactivate when a person is run down.

Human herpes virus-6 (HHV-6)

The HHV-6, as it is commonly known, is a relatively newly discovered virus and is also a member of the herpes family, causing swollen glands, extreme exhaustion and sore throats. First identified in the early 1980s, the HHV-6, like the EBV, exists in the bodies of those who are infected for life, but usually in a dormant, inactive form. Although more rarely mentioned in the scientific literature and widely unknown in the medical community, the HHV-6 is particularly nasty in that it destroys certain of the immune system chemicals (the natural killer cells) that are vital for maintaining good health. Furthermore, once natural killer cells are depleted, the door is left wide open for other viruses (such as the Epstein-Barr) to reactivate.

Cytomegalovirus

This is the most poorly understood member of the herpes family of viruses; however, it can, like the EBV and HHV-6, produce the chronic symptoms – sore throat, swollen glands and exhaustion – that are associated with CFS.

Testing for viruses

Life would be easy for CFS patients if testing for viruses was straightforward, but it is not. Although tests exist, the problem is with delineating between a recent, latent infection (one the body has already dealt with) and a reactivation of an old one.

When people find themselves initially infected, two immune-system defence mechanisms leap into action. The first is a set of virally fighting antibodies called immunoglobulin M (or IgM). These antibodies aggressively attack the virus and their levels will be at their highest for up to three months. After this point, the IgM levels will sharply decrease and a new set of antibodies or immunoglobulin G (IgG) step up to keep the infection in check, so that the virus doesn't reactivate. Because of this, IgG levels increase and remain high for life, since suppressing the virus is a permanent job of the immune system. So testing for viruses is tricky, since just about everyone in the population has been exposed to them and will, therefore, show a similar pattern of low IgM and high IgG levels, whether they have CFS or not.

This said, because viral infections are common in CFS and certainly many of the main symptoms of the disorder point to an ongoing immune activation, we cannot rule out a new or reactivated infection as the cause.

Other viral and bacterial infections

Although the herpes viruses, particularly EBV and, increasingly HHV-6, probably receive the most focus as potential CFS triggers, bacterial infections can also lead to the condition. In fact, you might have both viral and bacterial infections as underlying components of your CFS symptoms.

Here are some of the bacterial infections most widely associated with CFS:

- Barfonella – this is the name of the bacteria linked to cat-scratch fever.

- Brucellosis – most often associated with animals, this can also infect humans when they consume dairy goods which have not been pasteurised.

- Mycoplasma – this is a bacteria which causes a number of symptoms linked to lung (cough, pneumonia) and urinary tract infection.

- Parvovirus B19 – often a mild virus in children and adults, although some more serious implications can include anaemia, joint pain and nerve damage.

- Lyme disease – this is passed on to humans by the bites of ticks which normally live on deer and even sheep. One of the first signs is a bull's-eye-shaped rash and swollen lymph glands, leading to a wider range of flu-like symptoms. Hallucinations might also occur.

- Q fever – this is an exceptionally rare infection, caused by the bacteria *coxiella burnetii* and most likely to be found in Australian mammals, goats, sheep and cattle. It is normally transmitted through milk which has been infected and is usually limited to people who work with animals.

- Giardia – this bug can cause gastroenteritis, leading to diarrhoea, as a result of poor hygiene levels. Although mostly seen in people who have been visiting foreign countries, some domestic cases have also been noted.

- Hepatitis A, B, C, D and E – hepatitis, or inflammation of the liver, has also been implicated in CFS cases. It can be contracted through poor hygiene standards (A), exchange of bodily fluids (B), infected blood supplies (C) and other viruses (D and E).

The above are just a handful of conditions which can produce CFS or CFS-like symptoms. Obviously, if you have been diagnosed with a new viral or bacterial infection, have worked with animals, travelled abroad or have been at risk of hepatitis, your symptoms could be explained by these triggers.

Vaccinations

Although a small percentage of people seem to develop CFS following a number of different vaccinations, a firm link has not been established. Indeed, the possible connection receives little attention in the medical literature and remains a contentious issue. However, that some people might be susceptible to developing CFS following a vaccine injection makes sense, and is even a hypothesis pursued by Dr Charles Shepherd,[9] medical adviser to the British ME Association and himself a CFS sufferer. Given that vaccinations simulate an infectious agent so that the immune system manufactures the necessary antibodies to defend the body against a future attack, a vaccine might be 'the final straw' to an already stressed and overloaded system or an individual might have some kind of genetic inability to cope with that specific vaccine.

Environmental poisons and allergens

A growing area of interest in CFS research is the relationship between environmental factors, namely allergies, and toxic chemicals as triggers for the condition, or as the result of the body's malfunctioning.[10] Allergens, such as various pollens and animal fur dander and pollutants and other toxic substances, such as pesticides (especially organophosphates), mercury, lead, household paint, damp-proof treatments and poisons, may also strain the body, particularly the immune system, leading to an initial malfunction and inability to correct itself. In a similar reaction to viruses and bacteria, the immune system will identify these 'foreign' substances as threats and, as a result, organise an orchestrated assault on them. However, if the body is weakened, and therefore unable to fight off these invaders effectively, CFS symptoms can occur.

Psychological and physical trauma

People with fibromyalgia often report that their symptoms began following a physical or emotional trauma, such as a car accident, surgery or some kind of personal loss. The scientific literature on CFS rarely mentions such triggers, but they do occur. Although when we encounter emotional hard knocks we generally expect to experience psychological symptoms, such as sadness, anger or fear, researchers are now just starting to recognise the physical impact of such traumas on our health, i.e. that emotional setbacks can trigger serious physical illnesses. For example, in a study conducted by Dr Gwen Sprehn and her team,[11] it was found that divorce, in particular, leads to 'lingering, detrimental' impact on health for years to come, even if that person remarries and finds renewed happiness. Chronic conditions such as cancer, cardiovascular disease and diabetes, are some of the many debilitating illnesses following the emotional distress of divorce. Women experiencing prolonged social isolation and loneliness following divorce have been found to suffer an increase in breast cancer.

So difficult life events can cause us such distress and might on their own lead to a disruption of our normal, healthy immunological, nervous and hormone system functions. Then, because our body systems have gone into a state of shock and malfunction, old viruses, normally kept under wraps, reactivate. And because our bodies are unable to right themselves due to this widespread malfunction, further breakdown occurs, leading to CFS.

Body Breakdown

Irrespective of the many triggers, both physical and psychological, that lead to CFS, the body breaks down in response and is unable to right itself. There are undoubtedly infinite ways in which our body malfunctions when CFS strikes, but five main systems are affected:

1. The autonomic nervous system (ANS)
2. The hypothalamic–pituitary–adrenal (HPA) axis
3. The limbic system
4. The immune system
5. The gastro-intestinal system

As you read the following sections, you will notice that there are common symptoms of physiological breakdown. This is because all the above systems are interlinked, so if one goes haywire, there is a good chance that the others will too.

1. The autonomic nervous system

Whether it is confronted by a physical or psychological threat, the body produces the exact same chemicals in response. In other words, although the body recognises a general threat, it is not able to differentiate between the various types of dangers, and activates a very primitive response system called 'fight or flight'. This ancient survival mechanism is governed by the autonomic nervous system (ANS). The ANS, which also governs the hypothalamus (see p. 67), is essential to health and controls such vital functions as heart rate, blood pressure, breathing, body temperature, blood flow, sleep, vision and even production of saliva. All of these functions make up what we call the 'body clock', which runs on a twenty-four hour cycle. Sometimes this 'clock' is referred to as 'circadian rhythms'. Throughout this period, the body is awash with different hormones produced by our glands at regular, allotted intervals, keeping things functioning with sharp precision. Mostly, the process works like an efficient timepiece; however, it can be knocked out of sync fairly easily. Even just sleeping a couple of extra hours on weekends or pulling an all-nighter to study for exams can throw off the body's strictly honed hormonal production system leaving you feeling dreadful as a result.

The ANS breakdown can lead to the development of CFS. If you look back at the Canadian criteria (see pp. 21–4), you can see a number of wide-ranging and diverse symptoms, many of which can be explained by a dysfunctional ANS.

Many people with CFS suffer with one or more of the following and it is likely that a malfunction of the ANS is partly at fault:

- Immune-system function
- Body temperature
- Appetite
- Memory
- Cognitive performance
- Exhaustion
- Alertness
- Sleep disturbances
- Heart rate
- Vision
- Breathing

2. The hypothalamic–pituitary–adrenal (HPA) axis

Connected to the autonomic nervous system, the HPA axis is the gland master central to our body. For example, the hypothalamus, which is based in the brain, will send out important signals via an elaborate feedback system of chemical messengers, first to the pituitary (also in the brain) and to other glands. As a result, hormones in the reproductive organs, thyroid and adrenal glands all become stimulated. The hypothalamus, which acts a bit like an orchestra conductor or mission-control centre, is an active monitor, always serving to ensure the appropriate levels of hormone manufacture.

In my view, HPA axis malfunction is central to the development of CFS because the HPA is the cornerstone of good health, as you will see.

The following are some of the main signs of chronic HPA axis impairment. As with the ANS breakdown, many of the symptoms below are similar to those of CFS:

- Sleep disturbances
- Muscle ache
- Increased infections
- Hormonal production irregularities
- Impaired cardiac function
- Decreased liver function
- Increased sensitivity to stress
- Dizziness
- Low blood-sugar levels
- Postural hypotension
- Blood pressure irregularities
- Reduced production of cortisol
- Thyroid dysfunction
- Weakened immune function

When both the ANS and the HPA axis malfunction in CFS, it is likely due to burnout from trauma, viruses or stress. When you are stressed, for example, your hypothalamus normally sends certain signals (cortical-releasing hormone or CRH) to the pituitary gland to stimulate the production of adrenocorticotropic hormone (or ACTH). This, in turn, signals the adrenal glands to produce cortisol and adrenaline. In CFS, however, there appears to be a malfunction in the production of cortisol. The adrenal glands seem to 'dry up', leading to the reduction of cortisol and 'adrenal exhaustion'. When this happens, you become severely fatigued, your blood pressure drops and you experience immune-system suppression, leading to vulnerability to new viral attacks and reactivation of old, dormant viruses. There is also the onset of allergies and an increase in hypersensitivity to stress.

The interaction between stress, personal disease and ill health can also be witnessed by malfunctioning ANS reactions, leading to catastrophic body breakdown. When you experience psychological and physical traumas or even just the threat of one, your body leaps into action and produces the necessary chemicals to promote healing. This is part of the 'fight-or-flight' mechanism, which, as I said earlier, is our very primitive, innate survival response.

3. The limbic system

A part of the brain called the limbic system might also be implicated. The limbic system is essentially the home of our emotions, but it is also linked to both the hypothalamus and autonomic nervous system. This system also affects how we cope with stress (and most likely anxiety and panic), and is our primary mediating site when we are under threat. When this major brain region becomes weakened in some way, due to excessive mental or physical strain, infections, physical trauma (childbirth, surgery), emotional trauma, even child abuse, the limbic system also produces high levels of cortisol, which, in turn, could damage the system itself. An increase in emotional symptoms such as anxiety, depression, or panic could indicate a breakdown of limbic system function as a factor in CFS.

4. The immune system

Also linked very closely to the ANS and the HPA axis is the highly complex and multi-faceted immune system. In brief, it is the body's defence mechanism, keeping us healthy and fending off attacks from viruses or bacteria, illness and injury. If you envision your immune system as an army, then your immune-system cells may be thought of as soldiers, each with its own specific job to do. Some will identify and attack *any* foreign invader, while others will only target a specific enemy. When an infectious agent grabs hold, the infection site becomes a veritable war zone: the immune system kicks in, produces all kinds of cells, which first identify, then fight, then destroy and finally switch off when the job is done.

Viruses, as we have seen (see p. 60), can attack in different ways. In the case of stealth viruses they attack under the radar of the immune system, while old, dormant viruses can be reactivated when the immune system is sluggish and low. The way they thrive is by latching on to cells, invading them, taking over and reproducing their own DNA. Once inside your cells, these viral attackers effectively take over. Your immune system cannot at first fight the infectious attackers because they are lodged so deeply inside your cells that they are undetected by your immune system. In a biological 'cat and mouse' game, however, your body slowly begins to mount an attack. In response to the hijack, some of the infected cells will eject a portion of viral material outside the cells and, once ejected, the substance can then be identified and destroyed. This action is called a target immune response.

Antibodies are vital to the process of infection fighting, as they are chemicals produced by the immune system in response to an invader. Antibodies are made up of proteins and can be best thought of as 'keys' that fit into the 'lock' – or chemical markers on infectious cells. Antibodies also have a 'memory' in that once they have fought off a particular attacker they 'remember' the specific agent and destroy it immediately. When faced with an unknown infection, your body has to produce new and specific antibodies and this process can take some time. However, once your immune system develops the right 'key', its antibodies start to multiply with amazing speed, launching the attack and making you feel pretty dreadful in the process.

Immune System Breakdown and CFS

Here are some of the many ways in which specific aspects of the immune system breakdown in CFS.

Natural killer (NK) cells

We all possess, as part of our immune-system arsenal, natural killer cells, sometimes also referred to as NK cells or large granular lymphocytes. Studies have shown that many people with CFS have low levels of NK cells.[12] In fact, in Japan, CFS is often referred to as 'low natural-killer syndrome'. These cells have an instrumental role in fighting infections and destroying tumours. NK cells are also needed in the prevention of reactivation of the Epstein-Barr virus (see p. 61) and possibly CFS symptoms.

Cytokines

Literally meaning 'cell storm', cytokines are manufactured primarily by another collection of immune-system chemicals called 'T helper cells' and their role is to alert the body of an invader and then to help orchestrate the destruction of the infection.

Cytokines have aroused the interest of investigators of CFS, not only due to their role in fighting infection, but because they also interact with the hypothalamus and provoke many of the typical physiological effects of an activated immune system ('flu-like' symptoms – temperature changes, tiredness, low mood, altered sleep patterns, general achiness in joints and muscles). For the CFS patient, there is a problem with the body's ability to 'turn off' the system that fights infection, even when it is no longer needed. In other words, the 'On' switch remains stuck. In particular, it is the interleukins (a type of cytokine chemical) that interact with the hypothalamus, linking the HPA axis with the immune system. So if one breaks down, the whole chain of chemical networks is likely to be fractured. So this all links back to the biological causes perspective, in that, if extended periods of trauma or even a one-off personal upheaval blow the HPA axis off kilter, cytokine function can also be disrupted and become dysfunctional. Since cytokines are responsible for fighting infection, it might be that a dysregulation of the system means we cannot turn off the activated immune system, leading to chronic symptoms.

Another intriguing area of speculation involving the cytokines' role in CFS comes from a shift in immune-system function. Normally, when the immune system is functioning well, the

T helper I (TH1 cells) produce cytokines. However, researchers argue that there might be some shift to T helper 2 (TH2) cell cytokine production.[13] TH2 cells are designed to support TH1 cells and act essentially as boosters. But when T helper 2 cells take over and flourish, the immune system becomes dysfunctional. This process is precisely what happens when you have an allergy attack: your TH2 cells become hyper-vigilant and inflamed in order to fight substances (allergens) that are ordinarily harmless to the body. The TH2 cells don't recognise the lack of threat and create the immune activation reactions – sneezing, runny nose, headaches, etc. With a viral infection, it might be that the TH2 switch takes over.[14]

This abnormal immune-system functioning involving cytokines could also lead to dysregulation of the hypothalamus and other hormonal irregularities, triggering a reactivation of other infections.

So disturbance at the cytokine level would offer an explanation for both the 'flu-like' symptoms and persistent fatigue in CFS.

Lymphocytes

These are one of the main sources of attack your immune system has at its disposal. Composed of white blood cells (leukocytes) they are produced in the bone marrow. One set is called the B cells, which target specific foreign invaders, while another group travels to the thymus, where they develop into a diversity of subsets called T cells. It is these T cells which orchestrate the various aspects of defence, including the activation of the immune system, identifying and destroying the attackers, then switching off the immune system once the job is done. Investigators have shown that certain T cells, the CD4 cells (which act as body defence organisers) and CD8 cells (which suppress the immune system once the job is done) have been implicated in CFS.[15] Ongoing immune-system activation and, perhaps, the body's inability to shut the system off mean that symptoms of inflammation will still be experienced by someone with CFS.

Mitochondria

In every cell there are substances called mitochondria which provide energy – a bit like internal fuel pumps. Since our muscles and brains use the most energy, and because CFS has been linked to cell mitochondria abnormalities,[16] it should not be surprising that depletion of these energy factories leads to common symptoms such as cognitive impairment and achiness.

Although mitochondria can become dysregulated due to many causes (including the Epstein-Barr virus, see p. 61) the result in the body is chaos. Here are some of the symptoms of mitochondria depletion. How many do you recognise?

- Exhaustion
- Achiness in muscles
- Hypothalamic impairment
- Concentration disturbance, including brain fog
- Kidney impairment
- Heart function irregularities
- Impaired immune system
- Post-exertional malaise
- Allergies and environmental sensitivities

5. The gastro-intestinal system

Although the role of bad bacterial overgrowth in the gut remains controversial in CFS, with some healthcare professionals arguing it has no relevance at all,[17] others view it as central to the development of symptoms.[18] I personally feel it is highly relevant for many.

First of all, the gastro-intestinal tract provides an important immune-system function. Secondly, if the gut is blocked or clogged by excessive microbial growth, extracting important minerals and vitamins through digestion will be impaired, leaving the body essentially malnourished and lacking in energy. Also, many people develop CFS through overuse of antibiotics and can track the onset of their symptoms to use of these medications, and since antibiotics destroy 'good' bacteria that aid in digestion, this important facet of the immune system also needs to be addressed.

Candida, a type of bacterial overgrowth, can cause a wide range of symptoms throughout the body. Do any of the following apply to your health or lifestyle?

- Recurring bouts of sinusitis
- Mouth sores
- Long-term use of antibiotics
- A diet that is high in sugar or white flour
- Prolonged periods of stress
- Excessive alcohol
- Steroids
- Contraception pill or hormone replacement therapy
- Heightened emotional distress
- Exhaustion or lack of energy
- Bowel problems
- Itchiness, burning or discharges in vagina
- Skin rashes, eczema, itchiness
- Strong cravings for certain foods (alcohol, bread, chocolate)
- Headaches
- Symptom exacerbation in humid weather
- Memory impairment
- Indigestion and other digestive problems
- Sore or weak muscles
- Achy joints

- Fungal growth on toenails or ringworm
- Increased sensitivity to strong odours (perfume, tobacco smoke)
- Chronic ear infections or dizziness
- Numbness, tingling
- Anal surface irritation
- (In men) groin or genital discomfort, prostate problems
- Halitosis

Perhaps you don't think you have symptoms of Candida and none of the signs on the checklist rings true for you. Still, looking after your small intestine should increase mineral, vitamin and dietary absorption, leading to improved nourishment, stronger bodily function and recovery.

When the gut, specifically the small intestine, becomes imbalanced, this is often referred to as dysbiosis. In the process, certain micro-organisms in the intestines shift the balance, so that bad 'gut flora' or bacteria take over, possibly making you unwell. While many health practitioners nod their heads in agreement when asked about the links between CFS and Candida overgrowth, others completely dismiss the connection. And as with the many other debates around CFS, only time and more research will confirm who is right. In the meantime, let me explain the possible connection further.

Everyone has both good and bad bacteria, but mostly the balance is kept in check; however, Candida thrives on the organic material of the lining of the gut and, given the slightest opportunity, will reproduce and depress the immune system. As it flourishes, Candida can cause a whole host of debilitating and unpleasant symptoms (see above).

Medications

Another factor in the development of dysbiosis is the use of antibiotics. Even when prescribed appropriately for bacterial infections, these medications not only destroy the original infectious agent, but can also upset the delicate balance of good and bad bacteria.

Other medications can also encourage the overgrowth of Candida – steroids, the contraceptive pill, HRT – which also can themselves lead to immune-system suppression.

Since the colon is the host of yeast overgrowth, people often are plagued by symptoms typical of that area – constipation, abdominal discomfort, wind or diarrhoea. However, Candida can migrate to other parts of the body, heading south (to the anal regions) or north (to the oesophagus). It can also settle in other parts of the body – usually joints, muscles, throat, bronchial regions, urinary tract and skin.

'Leaky' gut

Candida is not the only gut problem people with CFS can suffer from. There might be a bacterial infection in the gastro-intestinal lining or you might be suffering from 'leaky' gut syndrome. This is said to occur when undigested food particles burrow their way through the intestinal lining, due to infections, parasites (including Candida and other fungi), certain over-the-counter drugs (such as aspirin and anti-inflammatory medications) and antibiotics, causing a breakdown between the intestinal tract and the bloodstream.[19] When particles of food – or other intestinal bacteria or toxins – enter the blood, they are then detected by the immune system as enemy invaders, leading to a variety of uncomfortable symptoms, including food sensitivity and intolerance. Since most people tend to eat the same foods over and over again, they might not realise they are placing further strain on their immune systems.

Cortisol

High levels of cortisol can affect the gastro-intestinal tract's important defence barriers by impacting on the body's ability to produce certain antibodies (called SIgA) which are found there. And if SIgA levels are decreased, the intestines become weak, vulnerable and less able to mount an attack against all kinds of invaders. Fungi, viruses, bacteria, allergies, toxins and parasites are then, as a result of this low immune function, able to enter the bloodstream.

So while we don't know what came first, the chicken or the egg, hypothalamic dysfunction seems to be at the heart of CFS. Our inability to handle stress further taxes the HPA and our immune system, triggering cytokines that, in turn, affect HPA functioning. In summary then, all roads seem to lead back to the hypothalamus.

By now it should be clear that emotional and physical stressors can place enormous strain on the body, leading effectively to a short circuit of the system.

The biological basis for CFS should also be apparent and, as an informed reader, you will now need to link your own symptoms to these biological explanations, because they are the theory that underpins the Fusion Model which you will read about in Section II. So take a few minutes to do this now before moving on to the next section where you will learn how to beat chronic fatigue for good

> **Marguerite**
>
> There was never any suggestion at all that my symptoms were anything other than psychological. Whenever I pointed out to my doctors that there had to be a physical cause because of all my physical symptoms and the virus I'd just had and couldn't shake off, I was dismissed as having a negative attitude. They kept insisting I was suffering from anxiety, despite my biological symptoms, like swollen glands and flu-like achiness. I was just written off completely and given no help whatsoever. It's only when I learned about the real causes of my illness that it all fell into place.

Julia

I knew I felt unwell for a long time, but because my symptoms were mainly emotional ones and forgetfulness, I was told I had a mental-health problem. It made sense at the time, but I was on a high dose of antidepressants which never worked for me at all. It was hell. I went to therapists and counsellors, but they never got to the heart of the matter. I felt abandoned. It was only when my brain started functioning again, allowing the antidepressants to kick in, that I was able to get relief.

SECTION II
THE FUSION MODEL: REPLENISHING BODY AND MIND

CHAPTER SIX

The Medical Option

I'm now going to introduce the treatment aspects of the Fusion Model. As I said earlier, the problem with CFS is essentially two-pronged: first there's the body's initial breakdown due to a specific trigger, then comes its inability to correct itself. Since the body simply cannot bounce back on its own, CFS patients often need help with this job. The Fusion Model in this section aims to do just that: replenish and strengthen the body so that it can heal itself.

We start here with the medical option, followed by the nutritional option in the next chapter. As each is a standalone approach and you will need to choose one or the other, have a read of both chapters before deciding which is right for you. Although there are strong overlaps between the two approaches, there are also some important differences – chiefly, that one is based on prescription medication and offers nutritional advice, whereas the other is solely nutritionally based; this merits careful consideration.

As stated earlier, both models cater for the huge range of symptoms and debilitation that characterises CFS. Although both are designed for you to follow at home, the medical model does require a willingness to take an active role in health management and symptom monitoring. If this is something you cannot or prefer not to take on, you should probably proceed to the nutritional model in the next chapter. Either way, remember these programmes have been carefully crafted by the respective medical and nutritional experts and must be followed exactly as spelled out.

Important Guidelines for the Medical Approach

Dr Mason Brown's medical model outlines four main easy-to-follow steps which you can undertake from the comfort and safety of your own home. However, before you even consider moving forward with this approach, you will need to look at the following guidelines:

- Consult your doctor, before embarking on this programme. It is important that you keep him or her informed of any changes you make to your healthcare regime.

- Read the entire book to ensure that your experiences of CFS are compatible with the views of the Fusion Model. The illness is so controversial and my perspective and that of the other highly skilled experts involved here challenges the standard treatment orthodoxy; because we are forging the way, with this pioneering and revolutionary recovery plan, our views are not mainstream.

- You could feel worse before you feel better. This is no small consideration for someone with CFS. Believe me, I understand this. If you are used to even a modicum of energy or independence, then a decrease in ability, even temporarily, even for the greater health goal, can be unsettling. Just remember, your body has been malfunctioning for a while, and many of the unpleasant symptoms you are currently experiencing are a direct result of this malfunction. So when your body is kickstarted into action, you can expect to feel an increase in symptoms – the flu-like signs, such as swollen glands, tiredness, achiness and emotional upset. This is actually a sign that your body is working again and is good news. Some people only experience a minor increase in symptoms; for others, like me, this is more severe. This is dependent on the length of time you have been ill, the severity of the viruses that triggered your illness and the degree of toxins that have built up. The difference is that now *you* are in control, so if your symptoms do increase, you simply lay off the programme for a day or two or until you feel up to resuming again.

- Different people heal at different rates. Don't be discouraged if a friend or a colleague appears to be charging ahead with recovery while you are still lying in bed. The end result is still the same. Give yourself healing time. Your job right now is to rest, look after yourself, and recover. That's it.

- Join a CFS support group in your local area (see Resources, p. 193) and go through this programme with some of the members. You can support each other all the way through.

- I would strongly advise that both you and your doctor consult Dr Mason Brown's website to maximise your healing success. In my experience, the advice offered there is invaluable. It will provide you with more background information on CFS and the man himself and offer you prescription medication advice. If, for any reason, you cannot obtain a prescription through your own GP, Dr Mason Brown or your local CFS group (see Resources, p. 193) should be able to advise you further.

- Follow the programme exactly as spelled out. As Dr Mason Brown told me: 'Getting better from this illness is like baking a cake. You have to use the right ingredients in the right amounts, in the right sequence, but in the correct way for you. Remember, everyone is different, so we do not respond in the same way, and we do not all progress at the same rate.' So don't do Step Four before Step Two!

- All supplement recommendations can be purchased from the stockists listed on p. 198.

Step One: Improving Brain and Body Circulation

You will need:

- Nimodipine (a prescription drug aimed to boost brain circulation – also known as Nimotop)
- Ginkgo biloba (to promote peripheral circulation)
- Eight glasses of filtered or bottled water per day (to flush out toxins and improve circulation)
- L-Glutamine (to promote brain function and general wellbeing)
- Evening primrose oil (to promote brain function and reduce muscle symptoms)

Nimodipine

We kickstart the healing process by 'rebooting' the body. At the core of this programme is the view that the vital brain functions – those which govern our body's health – are malfunctioning, leading to the bizarre array of symptoms that characterise CFS, as we have seen. The prescription drug Nimodipine (also known as Nimotop) is the cornerstone of this treatment and is the starting point of this plan.

Nimodipine is a calcium channel blocker, originally used with people who have had strokes. However, this protocol has been designed especially for CFS patients and the drug works in this context to eliminate brain toxins which have built up as part of the CFS disease process. Once these neurotoxins are reduced and then flushed out, your brain will function much better, because blood flow to the important gland master controls (the HPA axis) will increase. As a result, the healing mechanisms should then be switched back on, allowing your body to start to recover.

You will need to purchase a pill cutter for the Nimodipine (which comes in 30mg tablets). You can find one at any pharmacy. The dose required varies from person to person, but we all start with the same tiny amount: one quarter tablet.

It is best to take Nimodipine with food in the beginning because this slows down the rate of absorption and you want the process to be slow, so as not to strain your body. Also, try to take it at the same times every day.

Week one

Take one quarter tablet of Nimodipine in the morning and eight glasses of water per day. Do not be tempted to take more Nimodipine.

Week two

Continue taking one quarter tablet in the morning, but increase the dose by taking another quarter in the afternoon (preferably not after 4 p.m. as it can interfere with sleep). So you will now be taking a total of one half a tablet per day. Continue drinking the eight glasses of water and, as before, do not be tempted to increase the Nimodipine dose.

Week three

Increase your morning dose of Nimodipine to a total of one half a tablet, but continue taking the one quarter in the afternoon, so that you are now taking three quarters of a tablet per day. As always, drink the water and don't be tempted to increase the Nimodipine dose. This advice remains consistent throughout the whole programme.

Week four

While still taking one half a Nimodipine tablet in the morning, now increase your afternoon dose to one half. You are now taking a total of one full Nimodipine tablet a day. As always, drink your water quota.

Week five

Increase your morning dose of Nimodipine to three quarters of a tablet, but your afternoon dose of one half remains the same.

Use the above schedule as a guide: some people will need less Nimodipine, for example, a total of one tablet, while others might need more, say a total of two or even three tablets (maximum four).

However much Nimodipine you need – and how you will know this is explained in the box below – the instructions are the same: you start with just one quarter tablet and steadily and slowly build up. (**Note:** in some cases, the starting dose of a quarter tablet might be too much, in which case it's recommended either to begin with an eighth of a tablet or to take one quarter every two or three days.)

Essential protocol instructions

1. Always remember to drink the eight glasses of water a day and make sure it's bottled or filtered.

2. Do not increase the Nimodipine dosage more quickly than advised, no matter how impatient you are to progress. You must follow the protocol exactly as outlined. The key to the success of this treatment is its steadiness. Nimodipine flushes out neurotoxins and you don't want to overwhelm your body with these all at once, as it might not be strong enough yet to process them effectively.

3. You must monitor how you feel. If you experience mild facial flushing, headaches or nausea at any point, you have taken too much Nimodipine. If so, just cut back on your dosage, a quarter of a tablet at a time, until

those symptoms disappear, then use this as a starting point to build up the dose again slowly. If you experience these symptoms at the start of the programme, reduce the starting dosage to one eighth a tablet per day, slowly building up from there.

4. If you do take too much Nimodipine and experience severe facial flushing, for example, you can obtain another prescription drug from your doctor called Propranolol, which is a beta blocker. Dr Mason Brown recommends 40mg per episode to counteract any discomfort and the Nimodipine should also be reduced. This should not be needed if you follow the protocol exactly, but sometimes when people are too hasty and progress at a faster pace than is recommended, the minor symptoms of facial flushing, headache and nausea can become very uncomfortable. In such cases, the beta blockers should ease the symptoms.

5. Nimodipine is a temporary treatment. Some people only need it for a month or so, while others will need it for longer (four or five months at most).

6. If you begin your weekly increase and experience facial flushing or headaches which are mild, but noticeable, don't increase the dose for another week. Stay at the same dose for another week, then try again. If you continue to experience these symptoms, you will know that you have reached your maintenance dose and it's time to start reducing.

7. As you progress with the Nimodipine, you should experience an increase in cognitive and emotional function and a decrease in symptoms, including migraines. In other words, you should notice an improvement in brain function. This is how you will know you are improving.

8. At some point, you will reach a maximum maintenance dose and require no further increase in Nimodipine. You

will know you have reached this point when your brain and emotional functions have greatly improved and if, when trying to up your dose, you experience a slight headache (different from the usual CFS migraine; in my experience, neither severe nor disabling, but more like a niggle), mild facial flushing or increased heartbeat. These are signs that the Nimodipine has done its job and you should remain at the previous week's dosage.

9. At some point, this maintenance dose will itself cause the same telltale signs of taking too much. This is because your brain circulation is improving, the neurotoxins have been reduced and your body is healing. When this happens, begin reducing the dosage, by carefully reversing the protocol. So, say you have reached a dose of two tablets per day, you then reduce by taking one tablet in the morning, but three quarters of a tablet in the afternoon. Remain at this level until you again experience the indicators that it is time to reduce, and continue the process until you are no longer taking any Nimodipine.

10. Avoid grapefruit while taking Nimodipine as it interferes with the medication's effectiveness and always check with your doctor about other medication interactions.

This protocol is really very easy to follow. The programme has been designed specifically for people who are at home. The amount of Nimodipine taken is very small and the build-up is very slow so as to ensure minimal reactions. Just monitor your progress and pay attention to how you feel. You can always adjust the dosage accordingly.

You are now in charge of your recovery. Psychologically this is very important. CFS no longer controls you because you have the means to combat the illness. You can pace this treatment according to how you feel and this sense of empowerment should instil in you a sense of confidence.

Julia

For me, the symptoms were brain fog, brain fog, brain fog. I couldn't remember anything at all. I was also severely depressed. I could get around and even worked in a part-time job, but I felt tearful all the time and the world just seemed like one big blur to me. I was taking antidepressants, but they just didn't work for me, and that made me more depressed.

When I started taking the Nimodipine, after a couple of weeks I started to think more clearly and I felt stronger emotionally. I remember thinking, 'Ah, so this is how it feels when the antidepressants actually work'. The good news is, I was never depressed in the first place, it was all CFS. Most of my symptoms were brain related and one by one they all cleared up. Once the Nimodipine did its job, I didn't even have to take antidepressants any more.

Ginkgo biloba

At the same time as you take the Nimodipine, you can also begin taking the following supplements, starting with ginkgo biloba.

Ginkgo biloba is a popular health-food supplement. It is thought to help increase peripheral circulation (i.e. to the body's extremities, such as hands and feet). Take one 400mg capsule of gingko biloba per day. This dosage level is safe; however, if you experience any bruising, which is a known (but rare) side effect, you must stop taking it.

L-Glutamine

L-Glutamine is an amino acid that is an important source of energy for the brain. It also works to improve digestive tract function. Take one 500mg capsule three times a day for a month, after which you reduce to twice a day for one month. After that, a maintenance dose of one 500mg tablet a day is advisable.

Evening primrose oil

Evening primrose oil helps brain and muscle symptoms because it contains a substance called gamma-linolenic acid (GLA) which helps to relieve symptoms of pain, particularly muscle aches. The recommended dose is one 500mg capsule four times a day.

Step Two: Promoting Good Gut Health

This step runs concurrently with Step One. You will need:

- Prime Directive probiotic powder (to replenish good bacterial flora)

Probiotics

At the same time as you improve brain and body circulation, you will also need to tend to your gastro-intestinal tract functioning and start taking the probiotic. As we have seen earlier, many healthcare professionals acknowledge – although controversial – that a healthy gut is vital to a healthy body and mind. Since many people with CFS experience yeast overgrowth (also called dysbiosis, Candida, or bad bacteria) and this unhealthy balance can help prevent the absorption of vitamins and minerals, your digestive system needs to be addressed.

This programme recommends a probiotic powder called Prime Directive (see Resources, p. 198 for stockists) – it is an organic product and based on Dr Mason Brown's experience is most effective, but others are available in capsule form. (However, make sure you go for a good-quality probiotic capsule teeming with billions of micro-organisms.) Probiotics aim to replenish your digestive tract's supply of good bacteria and can also help improve symptoms of thrush, indigestion and irritable bowel.

For Prime Directive, the instructions are simple – you just mix the powder with water. You begin with a very small quantity, either one quarter or one half a teaspoon a day, either in the morning or last thing at night. It is very important that you begin with a small dose and build up to the recommended amount slowly and steadily. I cannot emphasise this point enough. By tending to your gastro-intestinal health in this manner, replenishing your stock of good bacteria, the bad bacteria will die off and be processed by the immune system. As a result of this immune-system interaction, you can expect to experience an increase in flu-like symptoms, such as tiredness, achiness, irritability and emotional upset. This is all normal, healthy and to be expected. However, because your body is still likely to be weakened and more fragile than that of a well person, you do not want to overload your system. You will have to gauge your symptoms here too. So if you do feel more tired than usual or other flu-like symptoms arise, either reduce your dose of Prime Directive or lay off the probiotics altogether for a day or two. This will give your body a chance to process the bad bacterial waste and eliminate it from your body. Once you start to notice an improvement in the way you feel, you can resume the probiotics.

Overall, you can expect to take Prime Directive for two to three months and then stop. However, I continue to take a probiotic every day as part of my daily health regime. Once, however, you begin to feel an increase in energy and a decrease in the flu-like symptoms, this means your body is now beginning to absorb better the vitamins and minerals in your diet. The energy from these nourishing substances is now finally reaching your cells.

Foods to avoid

Certain foods are known to encourage the growth of bad bacteria in our gut and should be eliminated from your diet. They probably include many of your favourite foods but, to paraphrase an aphorism from a well-known dieting organisation – *nothing tastes as good as energy feels*:

- White flour
- White rice
- Sugar
- Honey and syrups
- Stock cubes
- Yeast extracts, such as Marmite
- Soy sauce
- Smoked meats and fish
- Pickles and relishes
- Peanuts
- Mushrooms
- Any food containing vinegar, such as mayonnaise
- Chilli and curries
- Citrus fruits, particularly oranges, lemons and grapefruits
- Dried fruit
- Cheese
- Tinned foods and tinned juices

Foods to include in your diet

Once you have achieved good gut health, you want to ensure that the foods you choose also encourage the growth of good bacterial flora by providing the right environment for them to flourish. Here is a list of foods you should consider adding to your diet:

- Fresh vegetables and salad (organic)
- Avocados
- Seeds (e.g. sunflower, pumpkin and flax)
- Mild spices and herbs (e.g. oregano, basil, nutmeg, cinnamon)

- Herb teas and Rooibosch
- Cottage cheese
- Natural yoghurt from goat's or sheep's milk
- Rice cakes
- Soya and rice milk
- Organic chicken
- Fish (all kinds)
- Extra-virgin olive oil
- Artichokes
- Asparagus
- Bananas
- Buttermilk
- Endive
- Garlic
- Leeks
- Onions
- Shallots
- Tempeh (a fermented soya-bean product)

For more information on improving your digestive health, I recommend two excellent books: *Good Gut Healing* by Kathryn Marsden (Piatkus) and *The Beating Fatigue Handbook* by Erica White (Thorsons).

Step Three: Detoxifying the Body

You will need:

- Revenol (an antioxidant)
- Milk thistle (to boost liver function)

Once you have seen signs of improvement from the earlier two steps, and you are comfortable with moving on, it is time to begin Step Three which aims to detoxify the body. I would recommend that you wait around a month before you begin the detoxification process.

As you progress through Steps One and Two, always monitor how you feel. Once your neurotoxins have decreased, leading to improved cognitive function and your digestive tract has improved, leading to an increase in the absorption of minerals and vitamins, you should have reached a point where your body is feeling stronger. Throughout this process, always ask yourself how you are feeling. You and you alone, can monitor your body's response to each phase, so that you can tailor the programme according to your individual needs. This is not difficult, but it is essential, because only you can determine the rate of your own recovery. This is because, as we've seen, CFS is not a one-size-fits-all illness.

Your body will have been exposed to two types of toxins: internal (from cellular waste products) and external (pollutants, food additives and chemicals). Because your body has been malfunctioning, it has not been able to process these toxins efficiently, resulting in a build-up which we now need to address.

Revenol

Revenol (available at Neways – see Resources, p. 193 – and via the internet) is recommended for detoxification. Although there are other antioxidants on the market, I would always use this one for our purpose here. It is a capsule combining vitamin C, beta-carotene, and maritime pine bark. Despite its nutrient-enriched content, Revenol is a powerful detoxifying agent.

Detoxification should be undertaken very, very slowly because, again, the immune system will be responsible for processing these toxins. Also, you don't want to overload your body with excessive toxins, as this will put strain on your liver. This is why before you even begin considering detoxing your cells, you should wait until the 'die-off' reaction (see p. 111) from your digestive tract has subsided substantially because you can, again, feel a sharp increase in flu-like symptoms, especially tiredness, when you are detoxifying.

Some people only experience a mild increase in symptoms, while for others (myself included) this is more severe. Again, this is a healthy sign that your body is healing normally, but given the symptoms that are likely to occur, you should never push through the detoxification process. Slow, careful pacing is required.

As in the case of the Nimodipine, the starting dose of Revenol is very low. Unlike Nimodipine, however, you will not have to wait a week before increasing the dose. You can base your decision on how you feel.

You will need your pill cutter again. Begin with a quarter of a tablet. If you feel well, then increase the dose to one half a tablet the next day. You can continue in this way until you reach the product's recommended daily amount. If, at any time, you feel an excessive degree of tiredness or flu-like symptoms, then just stop taking the Revenol for a day or two, resuming when you feel better. Alternatively, you can space out the dosage, so that you take it one day, then have a day or two off. As Revenol is not a prescription drug, but is, in fact, a health supplement, you can continue taking it for as long as you want or need to, depending upon the detoxification process.

You will know that the detoxification has finished, because once all the toxins have been removed, your immune system is no longer activated in response. Any symptoms that you will have experienced such as tiredness, achiness and irritability will have disappeared as a result. Revenol has done its job once your body is functioning more fully and the nutrients from your diet are able to reach your cells – you can then expect to feel more energy, more vitality and greater wellness than you would ever have imagined.

For some, who have few built-up toxins, the process will be short. For others, it can be longer. I took Revenol for an entire year before I noticed any real improvement in my symptoms at all. This is because I had an extremely high concentration of toxins in my body. However, I can assure you, it was worth every moment because I have regained my health. And I would do it all over again.

Always remember to take Revenol after a meal, otherwise you might experience an upset stomach, due to the high concentration of vitamin C.

Milk thistle

While you are detoxifying you must also take a product called milk thistle, which contains a substance called silymarin. It is a popular supplement which can be obtained at any health-food shop and it is known to have liver-supporting properties. Your liver is your body's filter and, as such, is responsible for cleaning out toxins, so while you are undergoing a process of detoxification (meaning that more toxins will be pumped into your system), your liver will need more support than ever. Follow the recommended dose on the milk thistle bottle. You can continue taking it even after the detoxification process is complete (i.e. when you are no longer experiencing flu-like symptoms and instead feel an increase in energy) or you can choose to stop taking it once you no longer need Revenol.

Step Four: Replenishing Your Body

You will need:

- A high-quality multivitamin supplement (to support your body's need for replenishment during the recovery)

As you progress through Stages One to Three, your body will be working very hard to clear out the 'sludge' in your brain, gastro-intestinal tract and in your cells. Once these obstacles are removed, your body should now be in a more receptive state to accept all the health nutrients from your food. Because it has been effectively deprived of these nutrients (not necessarily because your diet has been poor, but because of all the obstacles to smooth functioning), your body will benefit from some additional support in the form of certain vitamins and minerals.

I would recommend a good multivitamin tablet (the Solgar and BioCare ranges are particularly good). Look for one that contains vitamins C, B-complex and E, as well as calcium, magnesium, zinc and selenium, and follow the recommended dosage on the bottle. You can continue taking the multivitamin as part of your daily dietary requirement or stop altogether when you feel well. Of course, I would also recommend that you eat a healthy diet (see Chapter Seven or consult a nutritionist).

The Recovery Process

As your body begins the healing process, you must rest in order to recuperate and recover. After a time, you should begin seeing the signs of healing. Your immune system will continue to remain activated, clearing out the sludge of toxins and dealing with any lingering viral infections which have placed added strain on your (formerly) beleaguered body. The process can take a while. The rule of thumb is this: if you have had CFS for up to five years, then expect to take a year to recover or at least improve your quality of life dramatically. If you have been suffering the ill effects of the condition for longer, anticipate a two-year recovery period. Your body has been through the wringer with a serious illness, so patience, perseverance and pacing are required.

Along the way, you should see evidence of major improvements, and with every new milestone – no matter how small in the beginning – you should feel victorious. Then, one day, after your newly healthy body has cleared the paths of toxins, the viruses have been sorted out and the flow of energy is now reaching your cells, thanks to a healthy gut and circulatory system, you should wake up with more vitality than you ever dreamed possible.

Think of recovery in stages as a progression: you start by embarking on the programme, then you notice improvements in your physical health; you then move on to the process of fitness and rehabilitation and, ultimately, you regain full health and re-engage with life as a healthy person.

Use the chart overleaf to monitor your progress throughout the recovery process. Rate your progress on a scale from one to 100 (where 0 = your worst symptoms and 100 = maximum health). Don't be alarmed if progress is slow; always remember that you are recovering from a serious illness and this is bound to take time.

	DAY 1	DAY 2	DAY 3	DAY 4	DAY 5	DAY 6	DAY 7
How am I feeling today generally?							
What are my cognitive symptoms?							
What are my emotions?							
What are my physical symptoms?							

In Conclusion

We would all like to bounce back as soon as possible, but your body can only heal itself at its own rate. During this time of recovery, you can expect to see small improvements along the way. Even the tiny achievements – making tea, going for a walk, sitting down in a restaurant or going out with friends – will take on new significance and be joyous events. So, remember:

1. Be patient.
2. Try not to worry or stress about your recovery time. It won't make your healing time any faster; in fact, psychological distress can delay the process.
3. Accept that you need time. Allow yourself to lie back, rest and heal. For right now, this is your job.
4. Always monitor your symptoms and pace yourself accordingly.
5. Always keep your doctor in the loop.
6. Use the mantra, 'Things must get worse before they can get better'. If you have flu-like symptoms it means your body is in the process of eliminating toxins and healing.

Marguerite

I was bedridden with CFS for a long, long time. I didn't need much Nimodipine because my mental abilities were generally OK, aside from some mild forgetfulness and I couldn't always follow complicated conversations or television plots. My real problem was toxins.

When I started taking Revenol, I really felt the reaction. I had to take to my bed, but then I learned to cut back and manage the dose. At first, I was anxious, because I thought I was having a setback. It really felt like a bad case of the flu. But looking back, to be honest, the symptoms weren't really that much worse than my illness was anyway. I was like this for a couple of months, then I started noticing I felt more energy. It was small at first, but definitely noticeable. The energy kept growing and growing and the tiredness and achiness eventually went away altogether.

Julia

You can have CFS for two years or you can have it for twenty. This is a serious illness, but how you deal with it is up to you. I didn't have many toxins and I barely remember taking the Revenol. The Nimodipine was the drug that really helped me. I remember going to visit a friend with CFS. She had consulted with her GP and the local hospital expert. She had followed their advice to exercise, exercise, exercise and she ended up bedridden. That is the difference I felt with this programme.

CHAPTER SEVEN

The Nutritional Option

Although the medical approach in the previous chapter is highly effective as the first step to strengthening the body, it's not for everyone. Some people feel that the independent nature of the programme is too demanding or they shy away from having to take and monitor prescription medication. If you fit into this category, there is another option for you – the nutritional method. You will still have to monitor your reactions and will still experience a die-off reaction (see p. 111), but this purely nutritional approach is a highly effective treatment for CFS.

Although I did not use this programme when I had CFS, mainly because I was not aware of it then, I can, however, recommend the two professionals who devised it. Alessandro Ferretti (Alex) and Jules Cattell are two highly qualified nutritionists who work in partnership and I have enormous respect for them. Through their understanding of the causes and nature of CFS they have designed an easy-to-follow programme, which you can undertake at home. Although they would recommend that you work with a nutritionist for support and to boost your chances of success, it is not absolutely necessary. (For more information about Alex and Jules, see Resources p. 193.)

The aim of this approach, which chimes in with the philosophy of the renowned American CFS medical expert, Dr Jacob Teitelbaum (see p. 54), is to nourish and heal the body through good food, dietary improvements and vitamin and mineral supplementation. There is also a strong overlap between this approach and Dr Mason Brown's method.

As always, consult your doctor before making any changes to your diet or health regime.

The Goal of the Nutritional Method

The nutritional model has been designed to reboot your body by building up and improving your:

- Immune system
- Gastro-intestinal function
- Circulation
- Adrenal function
- Cell mitochonsdria
- Liver function.

General Dietary Advice

We'll begin by making improvements to your food and diet. It might be a hackneyed expression, but when it comes to CFS, we really are what we eat. Food, diet and nutrition are the cornerstones of health and wellbeing, so it should come as no surprise to you that their role is essential in your recovery.

Many people with CFS have food imbalances, mainly blood-sugar dysregulation.[1] Their diets are often too low in protein and too high in carbohydrates, leading to a dysregulation of blood-sugar levels. It has been observed elsewhere that many people with CFS have problems with their blood-sugar levels. When we refer to blood sugar, we mean energy. So if your blood sugar is too low, you can experience many of the same symptoms associated with CFS – fatigue, weakness, headaches, emotional disturbances, dizziness, fainting (although just because you experience low blood sugar does not automatically mean you have CFS). Conversely, if you experience consistently very high levels of sugar in the blood, it could lead to the development of chronic conditions, such as diabetes, or throw your energy levels into a tailspin. So the aim here is to eat foods which carefully regulate your blood sugar and keep it well balanced. These should be foods that either release sugar slowly into your bloodstream or those which contain no sugar at all.

Blood-sugar levels often become dysregulated because of your diet. If you are experiencing low blood-sugar symptoms, for example, you might be tempted to turn to sweetened foods or caffeine, leading to a sharp rise in sugar levels in your system. This burst will quickly be followed by a crash, resulting once again in low blood sugar and its corresponding symptoms. The temptation is then to turn to the quick-fix foods (such as cakes, biscuits, caffeine), leading to a neverending cycle of boom and bust. Regulating your blood sugar will mean that you'll feel more energised.

To improve your health and vitality, it is recommended that you adopt a 'hunter-gatherer' approach to food. Use the following guidelines which will keep your blood sugar on an even keel, and set you up for life:

- Lean protein at every meal (chicken, game, fish – especially oily varieties, some organic red meat, eggs, tofu/tempeh, fresh nuts and seeds.
- Few or no grains (wheat, oats, rye) – they can stress the intestinal tract.
- Plenty of green vegetables/salad.
- Water, Rooibosch and herbal teas to replace caffeinated tea, coffee, fizzy drinks and alcohol.
- Aim for a ratio of one third protein to two thirds carbohydrates at every meal and for each snack. You don't have to be obsessive in terms of measuring out exact portions. It is roughly one handful of meat to two handfuls of vegetables.

Other good food guidelines

Here are some other tips to help regulate blood-sugar levels and give you more energy:

- Cut out all alcohol.
- Avoid drinks containing caffeine, such as tea, coffee, cola.
- Eliminate refined grains, such as cornflour, white rice, and white flour because they release sugar into the bloodstream very quickly.
- Avoid foods with chemicals, additives or preservatives.
- Stay away from foods containing sugar (including honey and malt).
- Aim to eat five small meals a day, rather than three large ones.
- Always have breakfast.
- Learn to cope with stress (see Chapter Ten), as people often turn to comfort eating and choose refined carbohydrates for an emotional boost.
- Eat whole grains – whole brown rice, maize meal and wholewheat pasta.

Essential Protocol Instructions

As with the medical model, the nutritional option specifies a special cocktail of essential vitamins and minerals to reboot your body into action. If you have been ill with CFS for some time, your body will likely have been denied the nutrients it needs for healthy functioning. While the 'hunter-gatherer' approach to food is the first step to a nutritious lifestyle, you will also need to boost your system with dietary supplements.

Some of the supplements used here are the same as those recommended in the last chapter; others are different. You can carry on taking the supplements indefinitely at the recommended dosage, once your body has stabilised or you can stop altogether when you feel better.

Before I detail the specific CFS formula, there are eight key points you will need to remember:

1. **For moderate sufferers** In general, always begin with the lowest dose possible for each product, unless otherwise specified below. The goal is to build up slowly to the full dose, depending on how you feel. I would introduce supplementation step-by-step. So on Day One, take all the supplements in Step One, on Day Two, add the additional supplements for Step Two, Day Three add the recommended supplementation for Step Three and so on. Keep going until you are taking all the supplements. You might want to spread out the process throughout the day; for example, taking half the supplements in the morning and the other half in the afternoon. Should you feel overwhelmed at any point, just cut back on the dosage or adopt a day-on, day-off policy.

2. **For severe sufferers** CFS can leave your body in a severely weakened state. If you are particularly fragile or frail, it is recommended that you introduce supplementation changes very, very slowly. To acclimatise your body and avoid placing your system under any further strain, you should consider starting with one supplement at a time, starting at the top of the list overleaf, then introduce an additional one every day. When you have reached the point when you are taking all the supplements, you might want to divide the programme so that you are taking half the vitamins and minerals in the morning and the other half in the afternoon.

3. Always monitor how you feel and track your progress using the chart on p. 98.

4. You could feel worse before you feel better. When the body is in a state of healing there is generally an increase in symptoms such as tiredness, swollen glands, fever, achiness. A lot of these symptoms are similar to those of CFS, but they are also a part of the normal recovery process, so don't panic. If, however,

these symptoms feel too strong, then just take a day off from treatment, maybe even two or three days off, resuming once the symptoms have subsided and you feel better.

5. The recommended products here are from the BioCare range (see Resources, p. 198 for stocklists), but you can find others at your local health-food store.

6. Start with the minimum dosage on the label and work your way up to the recommended daily amount. So, for example, if the label says, 'Take one tablet three times a day', begin with one tablet, then work up to the full three.

7. Contact your local CFS support group (see Resources, p. 193). Illness and recovery can be isolating experiences, so you might want to consider going through the process with others, providing each other with mutual encouragement.

8. If you are already taking vitamins and minerals, then make sure you don't duplicate. However, if you are taking something that you feel benefits you, carry on. If in doubt, contact your nutritionist.

The Supplementation Protocol

Essential vitamins and minerals

You will need:

- D-Ribose
- Acetyl L-carnitine
- St John's wort – but seek medical advice, especially if you are already taking antidepressants
- Whey protein powder

- Probiotic supplement
- L-Glutamine (1g, twice per day)
- Gingko biloba
- BioCare OxyB15
- Rhodiola
- Magnesium ascorbate (powder form)
- Phosphatidyl serine
- N-acetyl cysteine
- BioCare Vitaflavan
- Co-enzyme Q10
- Fish oil supplements, such as cod liver oil
- Milk thistle

Step One: Building Energy

Begin the supplementation process by taking the following energy-promoting substances:

- D-Ribose (5g, three times per day)
- Acetyl L-carnitine (1g, twice per day)
- St John's wort (500mg per day – but always seek your doctor's advice about this substance first, as it might interfere with antidepressants)

After you have taken these supplements, always monitor how you feel. If you feel well, better or notice no uncomfortable increase in symptoms, then proceed to Step Two. If there are problems, I would suggest going back and beginning with the first recommended supplement only. If no side effects are felt, go on to the next one and continue until you are able to isolate the supplement that is causing problems.

Step Two: Kickstarting the Immune System

Once you are ready to proceed, the next point to address is building up the immune system. Since the immune system goes haywire in CFS sufferers, you need to re-ignite it, restoring it to healthy functioning mode. To do so, take:

- Whey protein powder (the immune system needs protein to function well)

As we have seen, many people with CFS lack sufficient protein in their diets. This vital supplementation will help to redress this imbalance. Start with one scoop per day and, again, always monitor how you feel, regulating your supplementation accordingly.

Step Three: Boosting Good Gut Health

When you are ready to go on to Step Three, it means your body is coping well with the previous supplements, and is starting to become more receptive to healing. You can now consider improving the condition of the health of your gastro-intestinal tract. As we have seen, many people with CFS suffer from a malfunctioning digestive tract, either because it seems to be clogged with an unhealthy overgrowth of bad bacteria, leading to a malabsorption of nutrients or because a gastro-intestinal infection (a known trigger of CFS) preceded their illness. To address this you will need:

- A probiotic capsule, containing both *lactobacillus acidophilus* and *bifidobacterium bifidum* – look for a product that contains as many friendly bacteria as possible; each product is different, but the higher the content of micro-organisms, the better – aim for several billion

- L-Glutamine (1g, twice per day – a prime energy source to improve cell functioning in the gastro-intestinal tract)

The probiotic will help to re-establish a healthier gut lining. You can continue taking a probiotic every day as part of your health-care regime for life, or you can stop when you feel better. However, you should also consider taking pro-biotics if you:

- Have been taking antibiotics or are anticipating having to do so
- Are suffering from stress overload
- Have frequent infections
- Have long-term fungal infections on the nails or athlete's foot
- Suffer from poor digestion
- Are recovering from surgery or about to have an operation
- Suffer from cystitis.

Probiotic foods and diet guidelines

While probiotics are highly effective in promoting the growth of good bacterial flora, certain foods are also advisable to help nourish these friendly gut helpers. Try introducing some of these into your daily diet:

- Avocados
- Seeds (e.g. sunflower, pumpkin and flax)
- Mild spices and herbs (e.g. oregano, basil, nutmeg, cinnamon)
- Herb teas and Rooibosch
- Cottage cheese
- Natural yoghurt from goat's or sheep's milk
- Rice cakes

- Soya and rice milk
- Organic chicken
- Fish (all kinds)
- Extra-virgin olive oil
- Artichokes
- Asparagus
- Bananas
- Buttermilk
- Endives
- Garlic
- Leeks
- Onions
- Shallots
- Tempeh (a fermented soya-bean product)

Foods to avoid

As we saw in the previous chapter, there are certain foods which are known to help bad bacteria flourish in your gut. It is almost impossible to remove all of these substances from the diet entirely, however, it is worthwhile trying to avoid as many of these foods as possible:

- Alcohol
- White flour
- White rice
- Honey and syrups
- Stock cubes
- Yeast extracts, such as Marmite
- Soy sauce
- Smoked meats and fish
- Pickles and relishes

- Peanuts
- Mushrooms
- Any food containing vinegar, such as mayonnaise
- Chilli and curries
- Citrus fruits, particularly oranges, grapefruits and lemons
- Dried fruit
- Cheese
- Tinned foods and tinned juices
- Sugar

Die-off reaction

When the bad bacteria are destroyed, as we have seen, an increase in immune system or flu-like symptoms can occur as the immune system processes the dead organisms. This is referred to as a 'die-off' or 'Herxheimer's' reaction. The symptoms, although temporary, must be monitored very carefully, especially if you are very weak, and you must proceed slowly. Symptoms can be both physical and emotional, so watch out for a wide range of strong feelings. If even the lowest dose is producing a strong reaction, then alter the pace of your recovery. Remember, you are in control of your recovery and your symptoms. So, for example, instead of taking a probiotic capsule every day, make it every other day or every three days. When the symptoms reduce, you can slowly build up again.

Remember also that although symptoms can be unpleasant and seem overwhelming, they are signs that your body is starting to heal. Unfortunately, with CFS, you can become so clogged up with an overload of unhealthy organisms that a good clearout – albeit annoying – is necessary. However, once these obstacles to health are removed, your body will be more receptive to absorbing nutrients.

Step Four: Improving Circulation

A healthy blood flow is also essential to your recovery and that's what Step Four is about. Your circulation acts as your body's transport system. As we saw earlier (see pp. 26–7), poor circulation is the hallmark of CFS and many of its core symptoms develop as a result. So promoting good circulation will achieve two important goals: it will flush away the cellular waste products and toxins that have built up due to a sluggish blood flow and it will allow the good nutrients that energise the body to reach and feed the cells. To achieve all of this you should take:

- Gingko biloba (if you experience bruising, which can be a side effect, you must stop taking the product)
- BioCare Oxy B15 or any other antioxidant high in vitamins A, C and E

Step Five: Supporting Adrenal Function

Adrenal gland malfunction can lead to a number of CFS symptoms, including dizziness, fatigue, reduction in immune-system strength and a decreased ability to cope with stress. Your adrenals, therefore, need extra support for healthy hormone function and wellbeing. Again, remember to start off with the smallest dose of each product:

- Magnesium ascorbate (powder form)
- Rhodiola (helps to reset the body's reactions to stress, stimulates the hypothalamus and improves stamina. If Rhodiola is not effective, phosphatidyl serine can be taken as an alternative, see below)
- Phosphatidyl serine (can assist with resetting the body clock; this product is expensive and generally used as a last resort when Rhodiola is not effective enough. It can be purchased from BioCare and other vitamin stockists, see Resources, p. 193)

Step Six: Enhancing Mitochondria Function

The mitochondria are the cells' energy factory. People with CFS often have decreased mitochondrial function, leading to an elevation of symptoms, especially fatigue. The D-Ribose and the acetyl L-carnitine that you are already taking (see p. 107) help with this, as does the whey protein powder (see p. 108). However, to further improve mitochondrial function, take:

- N-acetyl cysteine (it boosts chemical glutathione – see box below – which is necessary for immune-system response and DNA repair)
- BioCare Vitaflavan or another antioxidant supplement (they protect mitochondria); check with your local health-food shop or nutritionist for alternative brands
- Co-enzyme Q10 (acts as your food supply's 'spark plug' because it releases maximum energy from it)
- Fish oil supplementation (1 tablet, twice per day – boosts concentration and improves cognitive function)

Glutathione

Glutathione is a protein consisting of three key amino acids: cysteine, glycine and glutamic acid. Glutathione serves many important health functions, including detoxification and immune-system aid and it boosts the body's cells' ability to reduce the damage of free radicals (toxic molecules which destroy cells).

Glutathione depletion has been detected in many people with CFS,[2] but healthy levels can be restored particularly through the use of antioxidant vitamins A, C and E and the mineral selenium. Foods containing high concentrations of sulphur, such as garlic and onions, and lycopene-rich foods, such as tomatoes and red fruits, are also powerful sources of antioxidants.

Step Seven: Supporting the Liver

The liver is the body's filter. Its job is to neutralise toxins, before they are further processed by the kidneys, the bowel and the pores of the skin. Everyone needs to support their liver function, but for someone with CFS, whose newly healthy body is coping with a backlog of toxins, this is even more important. The whey protein powder and the N-acetyl cysteine, which you are already taking (see above) are helping with this, but in addition you should take:

- Milk thistle (as directed on the label – also known as silymarin, it helps to support liver function)

Recovery Time

As your body begins to recover, you will probably feel an increase in symptoms. However, if you stick to the smallest doses of each product (spacing them out, if necessary, depending on how you feel), the discomfort should be minimal.

This nutritional programme aims to strengthen and heal the body, leading, ultimately, to an improvement in symptoms and recovery. Again, the method is not a magic bullet and the replenishing process can take from several months to a year, depending upon the severity of the illness and how well you stick to the programme. The process to recovery, in terms of stages, is similar to that observed with the medical approach, so I would recommend that you refer to the recovery guidelines on pp. 97–9.

While replenishing the body is essential to the recovery process, we also need to nourish the mind. Developing psychological robustness is the next focus of this programme.

CHAPTER EIGHT

Developing Psychological Hardiness

As well as being a physical illness, CFS also involves psychological factors. So while the medical and nutritional treatments outlined in previous chapters aim to stabilise your body and promote physical healing, you will also need to attend to your psychological needs, particularly your ability to cope with stress. If you don't address the emotional triggers of your illness and its maintaining stressors, you will probably experience only small improvements in your condition and are also likely to be more prone to relapse.

To this end, I have designed the psychological part of the Fusion Model. It is a programme of therapy which will provide the emotional support you need to boost your wellbeing. Throughout the course of your recovery and beyond, this programme is flexible and will help you to better understand the challenges you will face during recovery and after. It will provide you with the basics to motivate and support yourself and teach you to identify and tackle the stressors in your life, so that you can cope with them more effectively. However, if you feel overwhelmed at any time or are struggling emotionally, you should contact your doctor immediately.

Cognitive Behavioural Therapy and CFS

At the heart of my psychological programme for CFS lies cognitive behavioural therapy (CBT). Used appropriately, this method is highly effective and can greatly enhance your sense of control over your health and your life. However, the problem with CBT in current CFS treatment orthodoxy is that it is not used in the correct way.

Introducing the 'big five'

In some traditional therapies, psychologists teach people to overcome their problems by helping them to identify and better understand the link between their thoughts and their emotions only. For me, however, beginning on the psychological path to wellness means first learning about how we interact with what I call the 'big five':

- Thoughts
- Emotions
- Environment
- Physiology
- Behaviours

Each of the big five influences the way in which we feel, think and act. So in order to gain and maintain a healthy outlook on life, the first step is to grasp these different interconnecting factors.

Emotions and thoughts

People with CFS are no strangers to unpleasant, often terrifying emotions. Hopelessness. Despair. Anger. Guilt. Anxiety. They all go hand in hand with a devastating chronic illness. And, what's worse, thoughts tend to fuel the fires of underlying distress, which in turn, magnify the potency of disturbed cognitions. In a process I call thought spiralling, you can quickly become so overwhelmed by the magnitude of toxic thoughts that you are barely capable of functioning. This process is not only emotionally challenging, but also physically exhausting, made worse still by the fact that in many cases negative thoughts produce strong physical feelings, which almost inevitably lead to stress and cortisol production.

Environment and thoughts

There's no doubt that environment influences who we are. This includes our physical surroundings (such as the types of homes we live in and our workplace), as well as the people around us – parents, teachers, siblings, friends, lovers, strangers. All of these have the power to shape our lives in all kinds of ways, many of which may remain subconscious.

With CFS, the majority of people experience stress both as a trigger to the illness and following the development of symptoms, so the toxicity, pressure, constant demands have all shaped the course of the illness. Take a look at the environmental stressors that triggered your illness; you probably thought at the time, you had to keep going no matter what, juggling several balls and spinning endless plates, irrespective of how burnt out you'd been feeling. Maybe you didn't even realise your lifestyle was so toxic. Learning to recognise your limitations is essential in order to achieve and maintain recovery. You might even have to reassess your role and your beliefs about any 'super mum/boss/carer' image of yourself.

Physiology and thoughts

Life's irritations or annoyances affect the way that people feel physically – their stomach feels knotted, their heads hurt, they experience problems concentrating. And with CFS, this link is even stronger: when you don't have the strength to function very well, you cannot always think clearly either. Cognitive impairment is a common feature in CFS and 'brain fog' (confusion, forgetfulness, feeling muddled) in particular. Learning to analyse the wide gamut of CFS symptoms that is reigning over your body will provide important clues, not only to help you manage stress levels, but also to improve your rate of recovery. You will need to learn to recognise when you are overdoing it so as to avoid relapse.

Behaviours and thoughts

When a healthy person experiences psychological strain, they will notice some alteration in their behaviour patterns. Those who are prone to a more negative outlook will stay in bed all day and refuse to answer the phone. Others, with more angry ruminations, will lash out at loved ones or drown their sorrows in alcohol to take the sting out of their ire. With CFS, however, your thoughts also drive your behaviours. So you might close yourself off to the world because you are incapable of keeping up with social demands or are ashamed of your condition. You might not give yourself wholeheartedly to a treatment programme, because of past disasters. You might push yourself despite physical limitations, leading to an inevitable relapse.

Taking the big five exercise

Being able to analyse your thoughts, emotions, environment, physiology and behaviours will help you to build both physical and psychological hardiness. So I now want you to start thinking about your life in terms of the big five; because the more you familiarise yourself with these elements, the more you will recognise them and make appropriate vital adjustments in your life.

In the following exercise, look at each entry and decide which category – thought, emotion, environment, physiology or behaviour – it falls into (to get you on the right track, I've provided the answers to the first three):

1. Anger (emotion)
2. In the office (environment)
3. Argument with partner (behaviour)
4. Stomach ache
5. Sharing coffee with a friend
6. Excitement
7. Hanging around the train station

8. Beating heart
9. Bad things always happen to me
10. Mother-in-law comes to visit
11. Waiting for a job interview to start
12. Fury
13. Dizziness
14. My boss always complains about my work
15. Sunday afternoon
16. Joyfulness
17. I hope my presentation goes well
18. Adoration
19. Anticipation of a blind date
20. Doing aerobics
21. Driving the children to music lessons
22. Headache
23. Sweaty palms
24. Why do people always take advantage of me?
25. Misery
26. Dry mouth
27. I'll never be promoted
28. Resentfulness
29. My parents always loved my sister more
30. Insomnia
31. Avoiding a friend after an argument
32. Going for a long walk
33. Society is obsessed with youth
34. Apathy
35. Drinking alcohol
36. Doing yoga

37. Irritability
38. Slamming down the phone
39. Giving partners the silent treatment
40. Tingly fingers

How did you do?

You'll find the answers in Appendix B, p. 191. If you did well, that's great; if not, don't worry. Exercises like this can take a lot of practice because you're training yourself to look at the world and your role in it in a new way. Don't give up. Just train yourself. For example, at some point in each day, take a random event and relate each of the big five to it, regardless of how momentous or otherwise the particular situation may be. What was happening? What physical symptoms, no matter how minor, did you notice? What thoughts sprang to mind? What about your emotions? And how did you behave as a result?

How 'faulty' thoughts influence health

At the core of our psychological distress is what is known in CBT as 'faulty thinking' or emotional reasoning. When emotions spiral out of control, they influence the way in which we think, feel and behave, so that we are no longer calm or thinking rationally. The secret is to learn how to recognise faulty thinking, then to step back, take a detached view of the situation, appraise our perceptions of it and, as a result, come up with a more accurate assessment of what is happening. Here are some of the more common examples of faulty thinking – see how many you recognise:

Black-and-white thinking

This thought distortion occurs when we adopt polarised, 'either/or' patterns of cognition, so that something is either 100 per cent right or totally wrong. If your thought processes automatically turn to words like 'all', 'never', 'always', 'none', 'everything' and 'nothing', you are probably a black-and-white type of reasoner.

In the context of CFS, a tendency towards black-and-white thinking might turn into something along the lines of 'I'm completely useless now that I have CFS' or 'I have nothing to offer my family because I am so ill'. Destructive thought patterns such as these will only drag you down and cause you more distress. I know as well as you do that CFS can take over your body, your life, your existence, and reduce even the healthiest people to mere shadows of their former selves, but no one is 'completely useless' – we all have something to offer, even if our abilities are reduced. You are now on the road to improving your health, so when these thoughts/fears prick your beleaguered sense of self, remind yourself of all the things – however small – you have still been able to do while ill. Then also remind yourself of all the signs of recovery as you begin to notice them.

Magnification/minimisation

When someone has CFS, and suddenly even making a cup of tea seems like the challenge of the century, feelings of distress are understandable. However, people often magnify all their 'can't' and minimise their 'can' feelings. When I had CFS, I used to lament that I could no longer walk, whereas before, I was darting about all over the country. It was a huge blow. There are a lot of can'ts and not many cans. However, when you start nay-saying, remember that you are now on a better path and that these proportions will reverse.

Personalising

When CFS strikes, life changes beyond recognition. Many sufferers have to rely on others to perform even the most basic of tasks and this is a huge blow to the ego. Guilt, frustration, fear of being a burden and self-blame are just some of the many negative ways the illness is personalised.

You might resent others for not helping you enough or for not recognising how desperate you feel; you might even blame them for piling so much responsibility on you that your body burnt out in the first place. However, personalising, or blaming yourself or others is not only unhelpful – it is wrong. No one is to blame for

CFS. Sometimes, for whatever reason, 'shit happens'. And while you cannot change the past, you are, however, now taking steps to improve your health and restore the quality of your life. You are taking charge. So, if you do want to personalise, make sure you cast yourself not as a passive victim, but as an active participant in your own health management.

Jumping to conclusions

Many people react irrationally to situations, especially when they are already in an agitated state, often leaping to conclusions, even in the face of very limited evidence. With CFS, this tendency is very common indeed. Hopes are so often raised and dashed, especially in terms of progress, recovery or new treatment, that you may find you are often suspicious and doubtful that anything will work, becoming almost afraid to try. So you tell yourself that there is little point in attempting anything new and you look for evidence, no matter how scanty, to prove yourself right. I understand the need to be protective and avoid setting yourself up for more failure or disappointment. However, it is important to learn how to assess the quality of the evidence presented to you. Only once you can do this will you be able to have more confidence in the conclusions you draw.

Catastrophising

This is the 'doom-and-gloom/I-told-you-so' scenario: 'No matter what I do, it will end up in tears'; 'There is no point in trying'; 'Nothing ever works'. With CFS, there is usually a history of disappointment and false starts and I have found that catastrophising often occurs in the wake of a setback. It is usually an ego-defence strategy, designed to protect from more hurt or distress – we don't want to get our hopes raised only to have them dashed again.

The key to overcoming catastrophising is planning. Accept that even healthy people experience illness, and if you come down with the flu or a bad cold, assess how long it normally takes you to recover and remind yourself of this in the future. Also, remind yourself that the aches and pains and fatigue are all the healthy signs of an efficient immune system doing its job.

Characteristics of faulty thinking

In order to be physically healthy, you need to be psychologically robust too. Learning to identify your negative thought patterns or faulty thinking is crucial to healing, because it will help you to alleviate stress and motivate you towards your goal. This is an ongoing process and one that will take a lot of practice, because you are teasing out processes that are deeply ingrained in the mind.

Faulty thinking tends to be:

* **Automatic** – you do not need to be consciously appraising situations or even be focusing on them; instead, they often appear out of the blue. Also, you might not even be specifically aware of your precise thoughts. Rather, they can affect you unconsciously, by producing an uneasy or anxious feeling.

* **A distorted picture of your situation** – and, as such, not often realistic. This is because your automatic beliefs tend to be intertwined with your feelings, leading to thought 'spiralling' (see p. 116), so that before you know it you've envisaged the worst-case scenario and leap to all kinds of anxiety-fuelled conclusions, without any valid evidence.

* **Feasible** – in other words, you accept it as true, without question. Remember, a thought is not a fact, which is why you need to appraise your beliefs, no matter how valid or conclusive they might initially appear to be.

* **Tenacious** – it tends to persist and needs to be constantly checked and challenged.

* **Ingrained** into our psyches unless challenged. You accept it as fact, even when there is no basis, and it then forms a permanent part of your world view.

Faulty thinking is pretty powerful and exerts a strong influence. Once you identify it, you can challenge it and come up with a more balanced, more rational, less anxiety-ridden assessment of your situation.

Key CFS facts: recognising what you're up against

A lot of people with CFS ask me what the difference is between helpful and unhelpful thoughts, given that the illness *is* dominated by quite of lot of genuine negativity. Unlike most CFS experts, I believe the illness is valid, biologically *and* psychologically driven and globally disabling. Furthermore, I believe it is possible to recover fully from the disorder using the Fusion Model. Along the way, that means looking at your health situation from all angles, *including* the negative. In this respect, I often find myself in conflict with other therapists who want to focus exclusively on the positive. But in my view, dismissing the negative is akin to both 'magical' thinking (pretending the situation is different) and denial (pretending the situation doesn't exist at all). So, before you attempt to tackle any unhealthy or unhelpful thought patterns, I think it's important that we first look at some facts:

- CFS is biological, with psychological components triggering and maintaining it.

- CFS is genuine; it is not imaginary.

- CFS is not merely a symptom of depression, a bid for sympathy or attention or an attempt to hibernate from society.

- There are doctors and psychologists who still believe there is no biological basis for the disorder.

- Compassion fatigue sets in with friends, relatives, bosses and health professionals, who also often hold prejudices about the legitimacy of the illness.

- When you are tired, you need to rest, not push yourself through the pain barrier.

- You are now in the process of healing; you are no longer

a CFS sufferer, but someone who is working to overcome a serious disorder and regain their life.

- CFS is an illness of relapses and remissions. At some point, even after a lengthy period of wellness, you might experience a relapse. This can be disappointing, but you should restart the programme and take a long, hard look at the possible reasons why your relapse might have occurred. Were you burning the candle at both ends? Were you becoming overcome with stress?

- Viruses, illnesses, emotional traumas happen to healthy people, so you can expect them to occur in your life too, during recovery and after.

- You have more control over your illness and your life now that you have decided to embark on this treatment programme. You are no longer a passive victim stuck in a rut of illness, pain and suffering. You have the mechanisms and the means with which to heal yourself.

- Remember that while your body is in a state of healing, you will probably feel more tired and more achy, and that this is normal – albeit unpleasant. Some people experience only minor symptoms, while others (myself included) experience a fuller flare-up. Once your body has healed itself, your energy levels will increase and you will feel revitalised.

- Life handed you a major setback when you contracted CFS. However, you will be a stronger, more capable person as a result. Let's face it. CFS is not for wimps!

Identifying automatic faulty thoughts

This section will help you identify those situations and circumstances that lead to the development of faulty thinking.

Whenever you have a strong, emotional reaction to an event or a memory, whether it comes seemingly out of nowhere or tied to a specific moment, this is a good indication of a negative automatic or faulty thought. So use your emotional reactions as a clue to identifying the beliefs that hold you back and cause you stress. I usually recommend writing them down and giving them an intensity rating from one to 100 (where 1 is the least severe and 100 is the most). You might want to keep a diary or notebook handy with the following template:

Date/time	Situation	Physical and emotional feelings (and rating)	Negative thoughts (and rating)	Balanced view

Context for automatic thoughts

In the first two columns in the left-hand side, write down the date and time of the triggering situation, immediately before you experienced your unsettling emotion, feeling or shift in mood. For example, your sibling might have called you and told you that you have been ill long enough and it is time to sort yourself out.

Physical and emotional feelings

Your physical symptoms might include tightening of your stomach, racing pulse, dizziness or general weakness. Some emotions that might come to mind could be anger, helplessness, sadness or guilt. Record the strong feelings the situation has evoked and rate them 0–100.

Writing down negative thoughts

Our automatic negative thoughts are often, by definition, subconscious, and therefore, not always easily identifiable. This task will probably require some perseverance, but do not give up; you will become quite proficient at it eventually. Some obvious candidates might be: 'I wish my family would understand I am genuinely ill'; 'No one ever supports me'; 'I am so worthless because I cannot live up to the expectations of my loved ones'. Record and rate your negative thoughts 0–100, as above.

The balanced view

In the final column I would like you to challenge these negative thoughts, by assessing their validity and accuracy. You do this first by examining the 'quality' of the evidence that brought you to your conclusion, by asking the following questions:

- What experiences do I have to demonstrate this thought is not 100 per cent true?
- If a relative or a friend held this particular view, what would I say to them?
- Am I shouldering the blame for something that isn't entirely my fault or a situation over which I have no control?
- Am I jumping to conclusions without examining enough of the evidence?
- Am I focusing too much on my weaknesses?
- Am I ignoring my strengths?
- Am I pushing myself too hard?
- Am I trying to get approval from someone I love or admire?
- If a colleague, friend or family member knew I held these concerns, what evidence would they come up with to contradict my beliefs?
- If this thought were true, what would be the worst-case scenario?
- Am I being impatient or frustrated by my lack of progress?
- In five years' time, would I be able to look at this situation differently?
- When I experienced a worry or setback like this before I had CFS what did I do to improve the situation?

- Am I wishing the situation to be different when I have no power at this moment to change it?
- Are my expectations of myself and others unrealistic?
- What other explanations could there be for my situation?
- Am I making mountains out of molehills?

Questions like these really help to challenge faulty thinking and to keep you calm. Stress and strong, negative emotion are the enemies of CFS, so the more you practise through challenging, the healthier physically and emotionally you will become.

Adopting a more rational view

Just writing your thought patterns down will have been very therapeutic as you have had to articulate the dark worries and fears that have been plaguing you. Now it's time to come up with alternative and valid explanations for your situation. The conclusions you reach now will be based on the questions we have just looked at for challenging disabling thoughts. Here are some examples:

Faulty view	Realistic view
My family doesn't understand I am genuinely ill.	My family might not understand what's going on, but I have friends with CFS who sympathise. My new doctor is also supportive. I have been able to turn to them for help.
No one ever supports me.	Actually, my parents have been very generous financially. An old friend came round to see me and offered to do my shopping. I do have some people I can rely on.
I am worthless because I struggle to cope.	Having a serious illness does not mean I am inferior. I did not ask for this to happen. I am not to blame.

Now take an example from your own situation and challenge your view of it in order to adopt a more rational one. Use the table above as a template.

Further tips for spotting faulty thinking

- Look out for 'should', 'ought' or 'must'; these are good, clear indicators of unhelpful thinking or faulty reasoning. For example, 'I should be better by now'; 'I ought to be helping my partner more'; 'I must be a real invalid, having to move home with my mother'.

- Don't expect to spot every kind of faulty-reasoning strategy. You might find that a common theme runs through your diary sheets. Perhaps you jump to conclusions on a regular basis or denigrate your achievements or define yourself by your illness. The more you become aware of your own personal thinking strategies, the better. Just remember, everyone is different.

- It might not always be easy or straightforward to find evidence to contradict your worrying thoughts. If you get stuck, put the exercise aside for a while and come back to it later. Sometimes, we get blocked cognitively, when we put pressure on ourselves to perform.

- Write all these thought challenges down in your diary or log book. At some point, this process will become like second nature to you. Also, the clearer your written record of your worries and concerns and the challenges to these anxieties, the more you can refer back to them as you advance in the recovery process. You will be able to measure not just your physical recovery but your psychological one too.

Always remind yourself of how well you've been able to cope with CFS. Other people may fail to understand the degree of suffering involved, but that does not mean it doesn't exist or that it is not valid. You have been through the wars and that requires true inner strength. Tell yourself every day, several times a day, how truly amazing you are to have coped for so long with such a devastating and debilitating disorder.

> **Marguerite**
>
> One of the things I learned that really helped with my recovery was how to handle my anxious thoughts. CFS destroyed my world, and I was scared for a long time. But I trained myself to only focus on the small signs of recovery in the beginning. Normally, I would just overlook the good and focus entirely on the bad. The breakthrough for me came when I recognised even the smallest steps towards recovery.

> **Julia**
>
> I was so forgetful so much of the time, and the struggle for me was putting too much pressure on myself, trying to remember what I was doing at any given moment. I learned to challenge my negative thoughts, to stop beating myself up and not to take the blame for an illness that wasn't my fault.

CHAPTER NINE

Formulating Empowering Beliefs

As you recover from CFS, your views about yourself, others, the world around you and the huge opportunities that could await you will change enormously. That's because your position is shifting from that of a patient disabled with CFS to a recovering patient to a patient no more. Each of these stages influences your belief systems and challenges your identity and sense of self.

Many people with CFS take a huge hammering when they first come down with the condition, as most – if not all – of life becomes unwelcome, alien, illness territory, not only in terms of the new-found physical debilitation, but also because of the psychological impact of becoming non-functioning members of society. There can be no preparation for this and I am constantly amazed by the way in which so many people with CFS cope with so much hardship. They never realise it themselves, however – mainly due to frequent suggestions that their illness is psychosomatic, that their degree of tiredness is not unusual or that they are simply lazy.

After a time it becomes difficult not to absorb all this negativity and incorporate it into your beliefs. But don't allow these negative attitudes to colour your view of yourself. You might have been unlucky in drawing the CFS straw, but you are doing your best to cope with something so extreme that at times it is beyond human comprehension. This takes extraordinary inner strength. You are not a victim; you are a survivor, even if, at this stage, you struggle to comb your hair, brush your teeth or walk more than a couple of steps.

As part of the Fusion Model, you have learned to identify and challenge the faulty thinking that has caused you psychological distress throughout your illness (see previous chapter). Your next job is to formulate a belief system that strengthens, supports and motivates you. As you make the transition from CFS sufferer to recovering convalescent to healthy or healthier person, I would like you to develop new, helpful, constructive beliefs about yourself as you proceed through each stage.

No matter how battered your beliefs are, the good news is that they can be changed and replaced with constructive, inspirational confidence-boosting attitudes that work in your favour, nourishing and building you up. Remember, just because you have self-limiting beliefs does not make them automatically true. A thought is not automatically a fact.

Note: if any of these exercises brings up unsettling or emotionally distressing information, you might want to contact your therapist or self-help group to help you sort through them. Sometimes, though, before we arrive at healthy attitudes, we do have to explore the miserable. Painful though it can be (usually it's just unsettling), the process is, ultimately, empowering. You're emerging from your chrysalis.

Changing Negative Beliefs

This is an exercise I use with all my patients. It's a great way of extracting your deepest thoughts and attitudes. It works by exploring the most remote corners of your subconscious.

Step one: accessing the subconscious

Accessing the subconscious – or thoughts just below conscious awareness – is the first step in identifying deeply held attitudes.

Since the subconscious is not easy to get into – although it becomes easier with more practice – brainstorming is a very useful tool as a first step. So right now, I'd like you to take a large piece of paper and write in the middle, in big letters: 'My attitudes about myself as a CFS patient'.

Next, set a timer for ten minutes. During this time, I want you to write down all your beliefs, perceptions, feelings (both physical and emotional) and other impressions about your experiences as a CFS patient. These beliefs do not have to be just limited to your views about yourself. You could also include your experiences with doctors, friends, loved ones, bosses, children and many others who have interacted with you as a CFS patient. Write it all down: the good, the bad, the amusing, the depressing, the silly, the painful, the inspirational. No matter what pops into your head, write it down.

Use the full allocated ten minutes. Even if you have run out of ideas after five or six minutes, keep up the exercise. (Also, your subconscious will carry on processing this brainstorming exercise even after you've completed it, so don't be surprised if more responses emerge later. You can always add them to your list.)

Try not to write down your emerging beliefs and attitudes in an orderly fashion – aim for creative chaos instead. The subconscious isn't a logical function. It is usually disordered, communicates in metaphor and is rarely logical. So try writing in big letters, using different coloured pens and various styles of handwriting (all of which help to access the subconscious), and use the full page.

Step two: reviewing your beliefs

Once the ten minutes have finished, review your beliefs and scratch out all those which don't really ring true for you. Some will resonate more with you than others and will more accurately reflect your true, inner belief state.

Next, I would like you to divide all your positive and negative beliefs into two separate groups. In each category, list them in order down the page, as this will make it easier for you to concentrate. Here, we can aim for organisation.

So your positive column might include:

- 'I might be disabled, but only ask for help if I really need it.'
- 'I always remember to ask my friends about their lives and show interest in what they are doing.'

- 'I manage to entertain myself and cope with long hours of loneliness on my own.'
- 'I manage to function within a very limited financial budget.'
- 'I keep in contact with the local self-help group and share information and provide support.'
- 'I thank the people who care for me and show my appreciation for all their help.'
- 'I am responsible for my illness and I do the best I can to cope.'
- 'I am more than a patient with CFS. I am a complete human being.'
- 'I deserve wellness.'

And the statements in your negative column might resemble these:

- 'I feel like a burden to my loved ones.'
- 'My doctor treats me like I am an idiot.'
- 'My mother keeps telling me I could do more if I wanted to; I'm just negative.'
- 'I will never get better.'
- 'I don't deserve to be this ill.'
- 'I will never get my job back.'
- 'I am struggling to cope with all this suffering.'
- 'I will always be an invalid.'
- 'I feel like a failure as a human being for allowing myself to get ill in the first place.'
- 'CFS is untreatable.'
- 'People think I'm boring.'
- 'I am completely useless as a human being.'
- 'I am inadequate as a mother and wife.'
- 'I am jealous of people who are healthy.'

Now comes the quality-control feature of this exercise. Place the positive beliefs in a file and refer back to them often. Next, look down the list of negative statements and weed out those that are the least reflective of your beliefs about yourself and CFS. Choose those that really hit you powerfully – the most poignant ones. You can have as many as you want, but some people find it easiest to work with about three or five.

Step three: promoting healthy beliefs

We're now going to work with three to five of the beliefs you identified at the end of the previous step (later you can take as many as you want).

On another sheet of paper, draw a line down the middle. On the left-hand side, write in big letters: 'limiting beliefs'. Below this heading, list your selected negative attitudes. On the right-hand side of the page, write the words, again in big letters: 'liberating beliefs'. The aim of this task is to help you begin the process of overcoming these negative cognitions and transforming them into healthy, constructive, empowering messages. So let's say that in your 'limiting beliefs' column, you recorded, for example, 'I will never get better', now turn to the 'liberating beliefs' side of the page and write down a new, self-affirming attitude, such as, 'This is a medical and psychological programme that has been designed specifically to treat my condition.' Similarly, change 'I am completely useless as a human being' to 'Being a patient does not make me useless. I am still a human being worthy of love, compassion and respect.'

Tips for transforming beliefs

When you transform your old, outdated, unhelpful views about your patient status, it is important that you keep certain key points in mind:

- Try to use similar language in both the limiting and liberating beliefs. So, 'I will never recover' becomes

'. . . working to help me recover'; and 'CFS is untreatable' becomes 'This programme has been designed specifically to treat my condition'.

- In your liberating beliefs column, always use language that is positively framed – so no negative words. This is because we are aiming to reach deep inside the subconscious and this part of our brain responds best to positive language.

- The subconscious responds best to simple, straightforward words; there is no need to write down grammatically perfect or complex sentences. So 'I will never get my job back' becomes 'My job right now is to recover from CFS. Once I feel well enough, then and only then can I explore my career options.'

Be sure to record all your new liberating beliefs in the right-hand column, directly across from your old, obsolete, limiting views. Once you have gone through each of your limiting beliefs and reframed them into healthy new ones, take your pen and physically cross out all the old, limiting beliefs. It is important that you actually do this, as it reinforces your transformation.

Step four: the power of metaphor

When working with the subconscious, logic does not apply; it simply does not work with this function of the brain. Rather, the subconscious tends to communicate with us using imagery. So metaphors are used in therapy all the time in order to ensure that your new liberating beliefs penetrate through to your subconscious, replacing the old images with newer ones.

To work through this part of the exercise, you will need to find a quiet place where you will be undisturbed for about twenty minutes or so. Now, take a look at the following passage, which illustrates your metaphor in action. Here, I often recommend that people record the information and play it back while they are sitting comfortably in their quiet place; it just makes the process easier (if you do record the passage, be sure to speak slowly, with frequent pauses and use soothing, relaxing tones):

I'd like you to sit comfortably in a chair with your eyes closed, feet a little apart and your hands relaxed and falling loosely in your lap. Even though your eyes are closed, keep your head facing forward so as not to strain your neck. (You can, of course, do the exercise lying down.)

Breathe in deeply through your nose and exhale through your mouth, four times. Very slowly, very relaxed. Breathe deeply and evenly.

Now, I want you to focus all your attention on your feet and visualise them. In your mind and without opening your eyes, once you can picture them, I want you physically to tense up all the muscles in your feet and visualise yourself as you are doing so. Keep them tense for about five seconds and then slowly relax them. Watch yourself in your mind's eye as you relax.

Next, I want you to concentrate on your calves. Imagine your calves in your mind's eye and physically tense those muscles for about five seconds, visualising yourself as you do so. Now let these muscles relax. Let all the tension melt away, fade away, envisioning your calves as you do so.

Breathe easily and just relax. Now concentrate on your thigh muscles. I want you to imagine yourself tensing these muscles as you do so. Now clench them tightly for about five seconds. Then relax them. Let all the stress and strain just fade away. Flow away. Float away.

Breathe easily and just relax.

Next, I want you to move up to your torso. Focus all your thoughts on this part of your body as you tense up the muscles really tightly. After five seconds, relax and let all the stress just flow away.

Now move up to your shoulders and neck. Tense them up tightly, watching yourself in your mind's eye as you do so.

When five seconds pass, relax. Just relax and stay quiet for a few seconds, breathing easily and calmly as you do so.

Now we're going to focus on your arms and hands. First tense up the top of your arms, then your forearms and then finally your hands and fingers. Tense them up tightly into fists, visualising yourself as you do this. After five seconds, relax your fists, then your forearms, then the top of your arms and let the tension flow away, watching yourself in your mind's eye as you do so.

Now that you are in a state of relaxation, I want you to visualise yourself somewhere in the natural world. This could be a forest or a beach or a beautiful garden – the choice is yours. You feel very safe and very secure. This is your special place. You feel comfortable and at peace here. So at ease with yourself and the world around you. You've never felt more relaxed, more calm, more serene.

As you stand basking in the peace of your tranquil surroundings, focus your mind's eye on the scene before you. Concentrate on what you see, the smells around you, the warmth of the sun on your back and the cool of a gentle, soothing breeze on your face. You are at total peace. You are more relaxed than you ever felt possible.

Now it is time for an exciting journey. While still focusing on the peace and calm you feel, and the sights and sounds and smells of your surroundings, you begin your journey and suddenly you notice up ahead that there is a little cottage. It's OK to approach the cottage. It's a safe place. It's a good place. Only good things happen to you here. In fact, the little house is so charming and so welcoming, you look forward to seeing what's inside. You hurry up the path to the front door, feeling the earth beneath your feet as you do so. There's a large red door with a big brass knocker right in the centre. You lift up the knocker to announce your arrival, but the door opens on its own. The atmosphere is calm, peaceful and you feel immediately at home. You enter the cottage feeling safe and relaxed.

Inside, in the centre of the room, you notice a wooden table. It is OK to approach the table and you walk over to it.

There's a big, leather book resting on top and a golden pen lying next to it. On the cover of this book, written in gold letters, you see the words: 'My Beliefs'. Go over to the book, pick it up and turn to the first page. Notice the smooth feel of the soft leather as you hold it in your hand.

As you focus all your attention on this page, you suddenly notice that all your old limiting beliefs about your illness are written down. In your mind's eye, pick up the pen that's lying next to the book and cross out those old beliefs. Cross them out so hard and so vigorously, that the page is covered in ink. So much so, that you can no longer make out any of the words or letters. Once you have done that, I want you to envision yourself tearing out this page, clearly imagining yourself as you grip the book, rip out the page and tear it to shreds.

As you're standing there holding the crumpled shreds of paper, you suddenly notice a small fire in the fireplace in the corner of the room. Imagine yourself walking over to the fire and throwing these bits of paper into the bright flames. Stand there for a few moments and watch the shreds dissolve into burning embers as they finally disappear into ash.

Now you can return your attention to the book. Once again, pick up the pen and, at the top of a fresh page, write the words: 'New liberating beliefs'. Imagine yourself as you do so, concentrating hard on and taking time over each letter, each word. Next, I want you to imagine yourself writing down all your new beliefs about your return to health. Write them down slowly. Write them down with care. Think about each of these new beliefs. Think about what your life is like now that you have new beliefs about recovering from CFS. Think about how much more healthy you are becoming and how much more rewarding your life now is. Focus on your sense of liberation, good health, joy, confidence, achievement and how much better life is to become, now that your old beliefs are consigned to the ashes in the fireplace. Really magnify, strengthen and enhance those wonderful feelings. Feel the power as you do so. Take a few seconds and focus on the new you, the enabled you.

Now you can turn around and leave the little cottage. Visualise yourself as you walk out of the door. The sun is shining brightly. The flowers are particularly fragrant. Your feelings of peace and wellbeing are greater than you ever dreamed possible. Enjoy these uplifting moments. Serene. Powerful. Full of health. Enjoy them for a few moments.

When you are ready, gently open your eyes. Remain seated for a few moments, then slowly rise from the chair, taking care as you do so.

This exercise will help to reinforce your new beliefs about wellness, but it is only the first step. The subconscious needs to be reminded over and over again of new beliefs, before the message gets through permanently. Try doing the exercise every day to make your new liberating beliefs readily accessible to you for a regular inspirational boost.

Towards a Healthier You

As your body heals itself, you can expect to experience, as I did, increased tiredness and other 'flu-like' symptoms, as we have already discussed. However, even if you expect them, they can still seem unnerving and you might return to your old disabling, fear-based belief patterns. Other limiting beliefs could also emerge, which could cause you unnecessary stress and setbacks – worries about relationships, financial setbacks or career prospects, for example.

To address these issues head on, I would like you to repeat the exercise and follow the exact same steps. The only difference now is that you will be focusing on those beliefs that destabilise your attitudes about your recovery. Some of the negative, limiting beliefs that emerge might be: 'I feel worse, so I must be getting worse'; or 'The recovery process is taking a long time'; or 'My body is so weak still, I will never be well again'. As you brainstorm, you might come up with such positive beliefs in the first instance as: 'I am getting better'; or 'My body is now healing'; or 'I am now getting my life back'.

Without a doubt, the recovery process for CFS can be a long one. However, you need to take into account how long it took your body to create the conditions necessary to develop the illness in the first place – say, years of stress, followed by a serious viral infection and the tendency to keep going, no matter what. You also have to consider the length of time you have been ill, which will impact on the time it will take for your body to heal. Also, everybody's circumstances are different, so don't expect to heal at the same rate as others. And remember that every day you are one day closer to regaining your health. No matter how long the process takes, let your new liberating beliefs reflect these realities, whether it takes three months, six months, a year or even two.

> **Marguerite**
>
> CFS made me feel really bad about myself. I felt completely useless and guilty all the time that I was so disabled and had to rely on others for just about everything. What liberated me was accepting that I wasn't to blame, that I wasn't just being negative or completely useless. In transforming my beliefs, I began to see myself as less of a victim.

> **Julia**
>
> I never really thought about the psychology of CFS before. I just thought it was a physical illness because I was so tired all the time. I could never remember anything either. Names of friends, even my address. I hadn't realised how imprisoned I had become or how limited my life was. This limited me as a person. When you have CFS, it is a struggle just to get through the day and survive. It was when I first began to see myself as a survivor and appreciated how much I had to cope with that I started to see that I could achieve anything.

SECTION III
RECOVERING FROM CFS: MANAGING YOUR LIFESTYLE

CHAPTER TEN

Coping with Stress

If you have CFS, stress is the enemy, and coping effectively with the stressors in your life is vital. A good gauge as to how stressed you are feeling is in the way you answer certain questions. For example, when you look at your life, do you say, 'I can and I want to' or do you posit the alternative, 'I can't and I don't want to'. Obviously, the former suggests a healthy lifestyle where you are on top of things. But if you tend to feel a greater rapport with the latter, you are in the stress danger zone and need immediate aid.

Destressing the Body

Whenever we are stressed, a number of symptoms occur, both psychological and physical, many of which are toxic to our health. These include feelings of irritation, anxiety, worry, headaches, sweaty palms and sleeplessness. While some people can cope with more stress than others (a high allostatic load – see p. 58), everyone can benefit from destressing. And, of course, with CFS, tackling stress is essential. So whether you are actively feeling stressed or not, it is always best to get into the habit of doing relaxation exercises.

Relaxation exercise

Relaxation exercises are an extremely effective method for reducing stress and, the more often you set aside time for them, the more you will feel their health-inducing benefits, throughout the day. The key here is consistency. You must set aside time every day to begin with, after which you can make it just three times a week or so. To maximise the benefits, incorporate the exercises into your daily routine, just as you do with brushing your teeth. Exercises such as the one that follows will also provide a mental distraction to help fill the empty hours during your recovery.

Many people like to read through the following script first and record it, so they can just sit back and follow the instructions. This is the best way. Just don't rush it; take regular pauses, so your body and mind can respond. Here's what you need to do:

1. Find a quiet room, where you will remain undisturbed for a good twenty minutes: make sure the temperature in the room is cool, so that the atmosphere isn't stuffy. Close the curtains or blinds, so that the room is not too bright, and don't forget to turn off your mobile. You are aiming for a cool, comfortable, relaxing atmosphere to start with. Some people prefer sitting in a chair (make sure your head and neck are supported). Others prefer lying down on their bed. Begin wherever you feel most comfortable. And remember to wear loose, unrestrictive clothing. Keep your hands loose at your sides, legs uncrossed.

2. Close your eyes gently, if you feel comfortable doing so, otherwise keep them open and find a place straight ahead – on the ceiling or the wall – on which to focus your gaze. Spend a few moments winding down, settling into relaxation. Breathe in slowly through your nose and exhale slowly through your mouth a couple of times. Focus all your attention on your breathing, keeping it slow and calm. Often when we first relax and empty our mind of conscious thoughts and distractions, a veritable flood of other images comes into our focus. Briefly acknowledge these images, but quickly refocus your attention on your breathing. Do not try to force the images out of your mind because the mere effort of doing so will only increase tension.

3. Now focus your imagination or your gaze – whatever you choose – on your toes and feet. As you do so,

tense your toes, feet and ankles. If you are still too weak, just imagine that you are doing so. Focus all your attention on this area of your body, tensing and then, after a few seconds, relaxing. Let all the tension drain away, leaving your toes and feet and ankles feeling relaxed.

4. Now move on to your calves. Keep your gaze or your imagination on this part of your body for a few seconds, breathing deeply, in and out, as you do so. Tense up your calf muscles and visualise yourself doing so; tense them tight – as tight as you can. Then relax, releasing all the stress. Feel the muscles lengthening and easing. Focus your attention here for a few moments. Breathe deeply, in and out, releasing all the tension and feeling more relaxed as you do so.

5. Next, focus your attention on your knees and thighs, breathing slowly in as you do so, then slowly exhaling. Tighten your knees now and your thighs and, again, visualise yourself doing this. Feel the tension and the tautness; hold them like this for a few seconds. Don't rush. Breathe in and breathe out, relaxing this area of your body as you do so, feeling the strain ease away. Direct your attention now to your relaxed knees and thigh muscles.

6. Direct your gaze upwards now, to your hips, buttocks and abdomen. Focus all your attention on this area for a few moments breathing in and out, in and out, as you do so. Now tighten (and visualise tightening) first your hips and buttocks, then your abdomen. Hold them tight; feel them really tight for a few seconds, focusing your gaze or your imagination on this area as you do so. Slowly relax them – first the abdomen, then the buttocks and finally the hips, breathing in, breathing out as you do so. Feel the tension and the strain drift away. Stay relaxed like this for a few moments, breathing in and breathing out as you do so.

7. Now move upwards once again, to your chest, upper arms, forearms, hands and fingers. Focus your attention on these areas, resting comfortably, breathing slowly and evenly as you do so. Slowly tighten your chest muscles, followed by your upper arms, then your forearms and finally your hands and fingers, visualising this all the while. Hold them tight; feel the tension. Keep them tight for a couple of moments, then slowly release the tension, first in your fingers, then in your hands, followed by your forearms, then your upper arms. Next, relax your chest muscles. Feel them all releasing the tension, relaxing, lengthening, lightening. Breathe in. Breathe out. Breathe in. Breathe out. Feel all the strain ebb away from your body, making you more and more relaxed as it does so.

    Take a few moments now to enjoy these feelings of relaxation, as you breathe in slowly and exhale slowly.

8. Now move up to the muscles in your neck, your face and your head. Focus your attention on these parts of your body, breathing in and breathing out as you do so. Slowly tighten your neck muscles, then those in your face and in your head, keeping them tight and taut for a few moments as you do so, visualising the process. Breathing in, then breathing out, slowly release your muscles, starting with your head, now your face, then your neck, breathing in, then breathing out as you do so.

9. Feel all the stress and strain flow away from your body as you are now in a complete state of relaxation. Focus your attention on your breathing, inhaling, then exhaling, slowly, evenly, calmly. Stay this way for as long as you like; then, when you are ready, slowly open your eyes.

After this relaxation exercise, take care standing up. You might feel a little dizzy or light-headed – as if you've just woken up from a nap. Resume your normal activities when you are ready, but try to maintain these calm, relaxed feelings throughout the day.

Learning to relax, although it sounds counterintuitive, can actually take a bit of practice, so do persist.

Soothing the Troubled Mind: Improving Sleep

'In a real dark night of the soul it is always three o'clock in the morning.' So said F. Scott Fitzgerald, perfectly describing that profoundly angst-ridden state of mind experienced by many people, not only those with CFS, when they wake up in the small hours of the night with worrying thoughts spinning around their heads, spiralling out of control. Panic ensues, because at that precise moment, they are worked up into a state, yet unable to do much about their situation because it is the middle of the night and they are not thinking clearly.

When you have CFS, you often have trouble sleeping or sleeping through the night because of an inability to shut off your mind, which seems to race without relief. Here are some tips to help you cope with this:

- Make sure your bed is comfortable – the mattress should be firm, but not too hard.

- Keep your bedroom well ventilated.

- Try to avoid emotionally charged conversations, arguments or heated phone calls before bedtime. They can upset you for hours or even days, as you tend to replay the exchange over and over again. And when you are ill, you don't have the physical and emotional reserves to cope well with unpleasant encounters. Of course, sometimes, they are unavoidable; so, if you know you are likely to have an unpleasant chat with someone, try to make it earlier in the day.

- Don't stress if you can't fall asleep; it will only make you more wakeful. Instead, try listening to the radio, or losing yourself in a good book.

- Chronic ill health in general and CFS, in particular, bring with them a lot of worries and stresses: financial concerns, relationship problems, pain, etc. Should these very real issues plague your mind at night, try getting up, going into another room and, if there is an especially pressing problem – an unexpected bill, for example – brainstorm all possible options, even the most outlandish ones. Be as creative as you can, if an obvious solution does not leap out straight away. Next, rank all the potential solutions in order (from the most viable to the least). You can then revisit and revise these options the next day.

- If insomnia is particularly overwhelming and is really affecting your life, speak to your doctor who might prescribe a low-dose antidepressant (such as Amitriptyline, which has a sedative effect) or a temporary course of sleeping pills. Your doctor should be aware of your involvement in this programme and advise and monitor you accordingly about the use of sleeping aids.

With chronic illness and debilitation come endless hours of inactivity and a big void which fills up with worrying thoughts and fears. Sometimes, at night, I used to wonder how I would get through yet another day of tedium and confinement. Here, as with all your other worries, it is important to remind yourself that your job right now is to heal and get well and you need all your strength and resources to achieve that goal. As you recover, you will be able to undertake more and more activities, re-engage in life and begin to make new plans. You are on the road to recovery; you are moving forward, even if the process is slow. Inactivity, boredom, solitary confinement should be temporary states. You should hopefully no longer be trapped in chronic illness and this should be comforting and reassuring.

Keeping an Active Mind

Everyone with CFS will recognise the spectre of boredom, with too much time on their hands.

As human beings, we are designed to engage in activities of all kinds, and we are programmed, through thousands of years of evolution, to feel bored when our current activity (or lack of) fails to excite us. Plus, faced with long stretches of unstructured time (as in the case of CFS), our minds tend to turn to worries and anxieties, leading, in turn, to stress. So when we are bored, we need to find something to do.

With CFS, the range of activities is limited, but it's essential to divert your attention and keep your mind actively engaged. My point is that, if you have a lengthy healing time ahead of you, it is important that you keep yourself calm, unstressed and involved in some kind of activity that will distract your thoughts. The radio, books, music, television and DVDs are a great way to help with this goal. Try to choose programmes or stories that are light, good-humoured and fun. Stay away from anything depressing!

Despite our best efforts, however, our thoughts do sometimes stray into the worrying arena of fear and anxiety, causing us distress. If this happens, don't ignore them, allowing them to fester or spiral out of control. Instead, face them head on. Here are some tips for dealing with different concerns:

Concerns about seeming lack of (or slow) progress

Some people zip along, while others, like me, progress at a snail's pace. But the end goal is the same. When these concerns rear their heads, keep a diary and record in it all the achievements you have made, no matter how mediocre they may seem, to remind yourself that even if you are not consciously aware of it, every day or every week, your body is still healing. While flu-like symptoms are signs, as we've seen, that your body is on the mend, they can still be a source of anxiety; repeat that mantra from earlier in the book as a reminder that you are moving in the right direction: 'Things must get worse before they can get better'.

Concerns about the future

Your job right now is to focus on the task of getting better. However, it won't hurt you to start drafting plans about what you would like to do once you have recovered – as long as they don't cause you stress. Perhaps you can call your boss and update him/her on your progress. Or, if that is no longer possible, you might want to come up with ideas about what you would like to do once you have recovered – many people with CFS decide on different career options altogether. Having one eye on the future is encouraging and psychologically healthy; just don't rush yourself.

Concerns about loneliness, isolation and re-entering the social world

Isolation is one of the more common and distressing aspects of CFS. Human beings are social animals and the near-solitary confinement can be hard to take. Some people advocate participating in the local self-help group and I would suggest getting together with a group to embark on the Fusion Model together, supporting each other for the duration. CFS is isolating enough and this distant treatment programme requires independence and dedication, which can be lonely. Working together, you can spur each other on. Just accept that people recover at different rates and refrain from turning it into a competition!

Concerns about taking on new activities or progressing to the next step

As you recover, you will be the best judge of how many new activities you can take on and when. It is easy to fall into a comfort zone and become anxious about taking the next leap. My advice is to work within your limits and gently expand. You will know if you have taken on too much, but the longer your body heals, the more inner physical and psychological strength you will have.

Once you've learned to relax your mind and keep it occupied with positive and empowering thoughts you will have taken another important step on the road to good health, as it will help to bolster your emotional health and reinforce your recovery efforts.

Marguerite

For me, the worst part was being housebound, with so many hours in the day to fill and not being able to do anything at all. I was so isolated and so alone which added to the distress I felt. I learned to focus on simple ways of distracting my mind, like watching TV and listening to the radio – anything to fill the void. Doing the relaxation exercises really helped too. They eased my mind. They made me feel calm and they taught me to let go. CFS is so stressful and I was so wound up by it all. It felt great to unwind and release all that tension.

Julia

My problem was with my thought processes all getting muddled up. It placed enormous strain on me that I couldn't remember what I was doing half the time. I tried so hard to appear normal that it caused a lot of distress. Then I gave myself permission to relax, go with the flow and not put pressure on myself. I just let myself chill out and recover.

CHAPTER ELEVEN

Getting Active, Getting Fit

Nourishing your body and your mind are the vital first two major steps in your recovery. They work in tandem, so strengthening one will lead to more robustness in the other. You will also need to begin building up your physical fitness, at some point, along with your strength and stamina. Like every other aspect of CFS, people with the illness vary enormously in terms of their fitness levels – some lead a near-full active life, while others are bedridden for an extended period of time. Some people are largely immobile for years, even decades. The good news is, however, that no matter how disabled you are, it is possible to regain quality of life if not a full recovery.

Before we start, there are some points you must first consider:

- CFS is a serious illness and the physical effects on the body are not to be underestimated, so always check with your doctor before embarking on any changes to your fitness regime. Hopefully, they can also refer you to a physiotherapist who will help guide and monitor your progress.

- You must determine your own rate of recovery. This is your body, your health. So don't allow anyone to push you further than you feel comfortable with – not your doctor, spouse, parent or boss. Usually, people mean well and try to be encouraging, but you and you alone know the pace that is best for you. So don't cave in to pressure, subtle or otherwise.

- Following on from that, don't be tempted to push *yourself* too hard either. Once you have regained some strength and energy, it can be tempting to 'run before you can walk', but you can cause yourself injury if your desires outpace your abilities.

- Be honest about your level of disability. We will look at this in more detail on pp. 156–9, but if you have been bedridden for a year, don't expect to go out and race around the block. You will only set yourself up for frustration and disappointment. To put things in perspective, at one point I was paralysed; now I walk six miles a day.

How to Get Active

The two main strategies I would like to recommend here are graded exercise therapy (or GET) and pacing.

Like CBT, GET is often inappropriately applied in cases of CFS, as we saw on pp. 51–3. In the throes of CFS, the body is medically and nutritionally ill prepared to take on exercise – it is like suggesting that someone embarks on a programme of physical training while suffering from a heart attack. However, now that your body is recovering and you feel stronger, you can begin to recondition your muscles.

The aim of GET is to help people to develop strength progressively and systematically. In other words, you begin at one level and methodically build up from there. You always move forwards – so, for example, in week one you walk down a flight of stairs, then week two, you walk down two flights of stairs and so on. GET has its advantages because you can easily chart your progress. The key to its success, however, is making sure your weekly targets are realistic.

Pacing is also a popular strategy in CFS fitness development. The approach is different from GET in that the targets are not so rigidly applied or adhered to. You work within your own fitness capabilities, largely depending upon how you feel. So, for example, the first day you might feel up to walking down, then up a flight of stairs, but the next day you might only feel you can manage half a flight. In my view, pacing is helpful when you are still in the throes of CFS or in the beginning stages of fitness training. Because you still have to conserve energy during these times, your body's recuperation abilities will be more limited. However, once your body has become sufficiently stabilised and strengthened and you are well enough to take on more demanding physical reconditioning, GET is probably the better strategy.

Getting Started

Many people ask me when they should begin their exercise regime or at what point they will be able to tell they are ready to start. Again, the answer will vary due to the nature of the illness and the range and severity of your symptoms. Usually, the tell-tale sign is simply that you begin to feel physically able to do more activity and that you suffer no post-exertional malaise as a result. Having said that, even if you are bedridden, there are still exercises you can do (see p. 161).

Defining your base rate

The first step in this aspect of the recovery process is to determine your base-rate abilities, i.e. your present fitness level. Below is a wide range of symptoms from full health to total disablement, with several stages in between. Read these categories and decide which best reflects your degree of ability right now:

- **No sign of ill-health at present** Have you been feeling healthy and robust for the past three-month period? If so, this means you will not have experienced any CFS symptoms, either after physical or mental exertion or when resting. You feel ready and able to resume your pre-illness lifestyle, including work or education.

- **Very mild symptoms** You would describe yourself as mainly healthy, but with the odd minor symptom returning. You are well enough to perform your daily tasks, including personal care. Your ability to walk or get around might be limited, but you feel you can return to work or education.

- **Generally mild symptoms** If you are in this category, you would describe your typical symptoms as mild when you have not engaged in an activity, but a slight relapse might occur pursuant to physical or mental activity. You need no help with your personal care or your other domestic tasks. Your mobility is sufficient that you are able to walk half a mile or so with few symptoms. You would feel strong enough to consider working or returning to education on a part-time basis.

- **Mild to moderate symptoms** You would describe your symptoms as mostly mild or moderate. In general, you are well enough to perform your personal-care tasks and your domestic responsibilities. You are able to go for a regular walk of a short duration. You might feel well enough to consider returning to part-time work or education, assistance with walking or concentration difficulties could be provided.

- **Stable moderate symptoms** Typically, you can perform most of your personal-care and domestic duties, but might need help with certain tasks, such as cooking. You might feel confident in taking on some moderate mental or physical exercise, but you are not yet ready to return to work or education for any reliable amount of time.

- **Unstable moderate symptoms** You would describe your symptoms as moderate for most or all of the day. Following physical or mental activity, you probably experience an increase in symptoms. You might not be strictly housebound, but your ability to get around is limited to walking a block or two. You probably need some assistance with your daily domestic duties and personal care. Resting is probably necessary at regular intervals. You do not feel well enough to return to your job or studies, but you could perform some household chores.

- **Moderate to severe symptoms** Mental or physical activity most likely leads to some degree of malaise or worsening of symptoms. You are not strictly housebound, but you tend to need considerable support or assistance when you leave your home. You probably require some degree of help with your domestic chores and personal care, but not all the time. You possibly need to take several rest breaks throughout the day and feel you cannot work or take up your studies at this time.

- **Severe symptoms** You would describe your symptoms as mainly severe. You are typically housebound and need assistance with your domestic tasks and personal care, much or all of the time. Your ability to move around is very limited and you are very likely to be relying on a wheelchair.

- **Highly severe symptoms** Your symptoms could be described as severe throughout the twenty-four hour period. You only have the capability to perform a small number of physical or mental activities and probably require a high degree of assistance and supervision. You are probably bedridden most of the time and typically reliant on wheelchair support. Your cognitive abilities are likely to be largely diminished.

- **Mostly disabled** You are confined to your bed most, if not all, of a twenty-four hour period and housebound. You require considerable help with your domestic duties and personal care because you are not able to carry out these responsibilities unaided.

- **Totally disabled** You are probably experiencing the most severe form of symptoms, pretty much all the time. You are typically bedridden throughout a twenty-four hour period and cannot live on your own. You undoubtedly need almost constant assistance for your personal-care and domestic duties.

Once you have formed an assessment of your current level of ability or disability, it is time to look at the specifics of your daily activities. We will use this knowledge as a base on which to build.

Using the template overleaf, I want you to complete daily diary sheets that document all your activities throughout the entire twenty-four hour period, starting from 7 a.m. This will give you a thorough picture of your own unique pattern of capability and a good insight into your energy high spots and low spots. I found, for example, that my better moments were in the morning, until about noon, after which my energy levels would just plummet and I would have to go to bed.

There is no need to go into too much detail; you just need to write in the bare basics.

Beginning Your Fitness Regime

Using your activity sheets as a guide, the first question to ask yourself is: am I able to cope well physically and emotionally with the demands of my current activities? If the answer to this question is, 'Yes', you can consider expanding your activities to include more. If, however, it is 'No', you need either to cut back to a level at which you feel in command of your physical and emotional wellbeing or maybe wait a little longer in the recovery process before you start to push yourself.

Your activity programme needs three key ingredients:

- Clarity – be very clear about your activity goals

- Consistency – ensure that your regime is regular

- Common sense – plan your regime according to your abilities and don't overdo it, to avoid boom and bust

Week beginning (date)

	Monday	Tuesday	Wednesday	Thursday	Friday	Saturday	Sunday
7–9 a.m.							
9–11 a.m.							
11–1 p.m.							
1–3 p.m.							
3–5 p.m.							
5–7 p.m.							
7–9 p.m.							
9–11 p.m.							
11–1 a.m.							
1–3 a.m.							
3–5 a.m.							
5–7 a.m.							

Remember, if you feel tired, you must rest! If you have a setback, analyse the reasons why and resume the medical and psychological methods.

Once you are ready to begin your new fitness programme, you must work well within feasible boundaries. I will demonstrate this by starting with advice to those people who are the most disabled. Even if you are relatively well and feel the advice does not apply to you, the template will be the same.

Advice for the more disabled

We've all got to start somewhere, and if you are very debilitated, you can still strengthen your body, even if you have not been able to leave bed at all or if you spend the greater part of your day lying down. Your muscles will no doubt be very weak and deconditioned, so you need to begin slowly. Start with simple exercises, like flexing and relaxing your feet. If you feel up to it, you can also squeeze and release the muscles around your knees, then squeezing and releasing the muscles around your hips. You can carry out these simple exercises at several points throughout the day. They are small, but significant and effective, and you will find that they help you build up strength and stamina fairly quickly.

Once you feel a little stronger, you can try sitting up in bed for a minute, then slowly, even if it is just by an additional minute or two a day, increase the amount of time you sit up. Always be cognisant of how you feel and the effects of the exercise on your body.

Next, you might want to try sitting up in a chair. In a similar fashion, depending on how you feel, you can start with as little as one minute, then build up, minute by minute every day. You will know you have done too much if you feel more tired. If so, just cut back.

Once you have managed ten minutes or so of sitting up in a chair, you can move on to standing up and walking a few steps. From your chair or your bed, you can start walking five paces forwards and five paces back. From this beginning point, you can again build on this success in a similar manner.

If your leg muscles are still really weak, you can build them up in other ways. I was so disabled, for example, I was not able to lift my legs up at all. They were too weak even to wear shoes, and I was unable to walk up even one step. To build up these muscles, I found a copy of a very thin, local telephone book and began stepping up on that. Slowly, I added more and more phone books, so that I could recondition my legs. Once I achieved this goal, I began to use the stairs, one step at a time, then one flight at a time, until I was able to walk up and down four flights of stairs.

As for your hands and arms, you can begin building up strength by using tins of baked beans as makeshift weights. Take one in each hand and, sitting down or standing, hold your arms straight out in front of you. Bend your elbows up towards your chest and bring the tins towards your shoulders. Start by doing this once, then build up slowly from there.

Here are some other activities of varying difficulty that you can try to do around the house to help you build up strength and fitness:

- Take a shower or bath
- Clear the table after dinner
- Help prepare a meal
- Dust
- Groom pets
- Put clothes in the washing machine
- Comb your hair
- Vacuum the carpet
- Put shopping away
- Write a letter

Progress might seem frustratingly slow. If you are severely debilitated, however, just keep reminding yourself of how much you have achieved, no matter how little. It took me six months to go from being totally bedridden to walking six miles a day. I gauged my progress and was able to achieve this amazing recovery because I never pushed myself, lost patience or gave up.

Advice for the more moderately able

The principles of building up strength, stamina and fitness are basically the same for you as they are for the more severely disabled. The idea is to build up slowly, methodically and to avoid any boom-and-bust behaviours.

Since you already possess a fairly high to very high degree of fitness, you have a solid repertoire on which to build. You could try, for example, going for a walk and increasing that distance incrementally. For example, you can begin by doing one block the first week, two blocks the second week and so on. If, however, you are not sufficiently challenged by these elementary activities, you could consider some of the following (however, just remember you might have to build up to these first):

- Water aerobics
- Pilates
- Outing to the cinema
- Meeting a friend for tea
- Walking your dog
- Going for a bike ride
- Horseriding
- Yoga
- Joining a book club
- Taking an evening class

The key is to find activities you enjoy which motivate you and help to build up your strength. No matter what your level of fitness is, however, you will have to keep monitoring your progress and making the necessary adjustments if you overdo it.

Advice for the more/fully able

As you are not bedridden or housebound and are probably already leading an active life, I would suggest only that you pare down your responsibilities and avoid taking on too much activity while you are following this programme.

Key points for getting active

- Always rest when you need to!
- Wear comfortable clothing.
- Ensure you can cope well with your current activity levels before moving on to the next step in your recovery programme.
- If you overdo it, take the next day (or couple of days) off and recover.

Tracking Your Progress

Using the target sheet opposite as a template, record your progress with your activity programme. It's a great reminder of just how far you have come as the weeks pass.

Your body is now becoming medically and nutritionally more stabilised and your belief systems are helping you to develop the essential psychological hardiness needed to persevere through what can be a lengthy process of recovery. Whenever you need motivation, just look back and see how much you have progressed from your days as a patient.

Target sheet

Activity	Monday	Tuesday	Wednesday	Thursday	Friday	Saturday	Sunday

Marguerite

CFS really weakened me. I was bedridden for months at a time; sometimes I even had to rely on a wheelchair. I eventually had to move back in with my parents. As soon as I got better, I would always rush around. I know I shouldn't have, but I did. I was just so thrilled to be able to see my friends, socialise and be human. Then the inevitable would happen and I would crash and burn. CFS would always win. I learned the hard way. I had to be sensible with my health, so I began to approach my recovery in a more sensible way. It was frustrating, but I built up my strength slowly. Baby steps all the way. It was slow, but as soon as I saw even little signs of fitness and strength, it motivated me to keep going. I am now back at work. And I never thought that this would happen.

Julia

I was never that badly off; not like most. I was never bedridden – usually only after a virus. I could always walk and worked part-time, but I was always stuck in a rut, always tired. I could never go on holiday or go to uni, but I still could look after myself. For me, the problems were with my memory. Then I started to remember things better and I felt stronger physically. The two things together gave me more confidence to be a little more adventurous. Sometimes I would overdo it, like stay up too late at a party, but I would just rest the next day. What I found was I didn't get that dreadful kickback after a couple of days like I always did. That awful aching and tiredness that would hit me two days later. I felt better and I started to trust my body more.

CHAPTER TWELVE
Dealing with Setbacks

CFS is a slippery eel of an illness, beset with remissions and relapses. Although you are now in the process of replenishing your body and your mind, and fortifying yourself against the factors that adversely affect your wellbeing, at some point, you might suffer a setback, if not a full-blown relapse. This vulnerability is in the ugly nature of the beast and you will have to look after your health for life as a result. This will, of course, be disappointing news. However, by accepting this basic fact about the illness right from the outset, you will hopefully be more conscious of looking after yourself physically and emotionally in order to prevent any slips.

The Most Common Causes of Relapse

The first step towards minimising your chances of a setback is to recognise the potential triggers of a relapse. The good news is that scientific literature has identified a number of the more common precipitating events.[1] They include:

- Surgery
- Anaesthetics
- Extreme changes in temperature
- Dental treatment
- Cold weather
- Chemicals (especially organophosphates, strong diesel and paint fumes)

- Physical trauma (accidents, childbirth)
- Changes in hormones following pregnancy or menopause
- Emotional trauma (divorce, job loss, death in the family)
- Viral or bacterial infection
- Excessive physical or mental exertion
- Poor nutrition
- Stress
- Immunisation

Many of these triggers will seem familiar to you by now. This is because the same factors that cause a relapse are often the very ones that set the ball rolling in the first place. So knowing what the triggers are likely to be gives you an advantage. Some are avoidable altogether, while with others (if you know that you have an upcoming operation, for example, or you are going through the miseries of a divorce) you will know to take especially good care of yourself, during that particularly turbulent time. Also, now that your body and mind are much stronger than they have been for a while, you should be more resilient and better armed to fend off any attack. As a result, the period of relapse should be shorter in duration and you can expect to regain your vitality more quickly. Finally, it is important to keep remembering that you are now in control of your illness. CFS no longer controls you, which, psychologically, is very important. In the past, CFS dominated your life, but you are now equipped with the tools designed to regain your health.

How to Deal with a Relapse

If you have a setback, immediately restart the course. So if you opted for the medical approach, resume the Nimodipine, the gingko biloba, etc. Similarly, if you adopted the nutritional method, begin following the advice in that programme too, as if for the first time.

We need to get you back on the right track as soon as possible, which also means eating a healthy diet and looking after your mental health. If you have taken on too much, now is the time to stop. You should not be rushing around like crazy; this will only make things worse. You will need to rest, recuperate, and resume the stress-management techniques (see Chapter Ten). Think tonic for the body; tonic for the mind.

Here are some guidelines:

- Inform your doctor. Always keep him or her in the loop.

- Relapses and remissions are characteristic of CFS. Don't deny a setback or pretend it's not happening. It won't go away by itself. Face it. Deal with it. Control it. Get rid of it. And get your life back.

- Don't beat yourself up. Of course it is disappointing and frustrating if CFS once again rears its ugly head. But instead of allowing these emotions to eat you up inside, learn from the situation. Ask yourself what the triggers were. Were you working too hard? Not looking after your health? Letting life's upsets chip away at you? Part of the process of recovery involves learning to trust your body's ability to heal itself: the more your body rights itself following a minor or even major setback the more this will strengthen your faith.

- Identify the coping strategies that work best for you and stick with them, even after you've recovered. Remember the old saying, 'An ounce of prevention is worth a pound of cure'? Post this all over your home if you have to, and make sure it becomes another personal mantra.

Keeping Your Immune System Fit

One way to strive for robustness and to minimise the likelihood of a setback is by ensuring that your immune system is functioning as efficiently as possible. The immune system is a vital part of your health, and its malfunction is, as we've seen, a major trigger for CFS symptoms (see pp. 25–6). These are some of the immune-system attackers:

- Sadness
- Negative attitudes and emotions, which are persistent
- Infectious illnesses
- Lack of or excessive exercise
- Poor nutrition
- Bodily trauma and accidents
- Over- or under-eating
- Food additives and chemicals
- Pollution
- Stress
- Smoking

We've established that recovery from CFS and maintaining your health means looking after yourself and taking good care for life. And, it is worth it. However, even with the best will in the world, sometimes we become lax, take our recovery for granted and return to old, bad habits.

To gauge whether you are guilty of this, look at the following questions; the more you answer 'Yes' to, the more likely it is that your immune system is under stress:

- Is your sleep regularly disturbed?
- Do you find yourself irritable and tense a lot of the time?
- Are you experiencing general achiness?
- Are you suffering from some other kind of illness?
- Does your diet consist mainly of junk food, convenience food or snacks?
- Do you infrequently consume fresh fruit and vegetables?

- Do you have difficulties with your weight, either with losing or gaining pounds?
- Are you experiencing symptoms of allergies?
- Do you rely on smoking, alcohol or caffeine to get you through the day?
- Do you rarely engage in exercise?
- Are you experiencing social isolation?
- Do you feel overwhelmed by life's pressures?
- Are you uncomfortable in the company of other people?
- Do you find it difficult to relax?
- Are you often exhausted?
- Are you frequently coming down with colds and flu?
- Are you finding difficulty in enjoying life?
- Are your concentration levels impaired?
- Do you snap at others for no reason?
- Do you have odd dreams?

These are all potential warning signs of immune depletion and if you notice more than a couple of changes, then your body and mind are providing you with vital warnings that something is not quite right.

Recipe for good health

With a history of CFS, it is vital that you look after your health and wellbeing. And it's not difficult:

1. Eat well.
2. Exercise regularly.
3. Don't take on too many responsibilities.
4. Get enough sleep.

5. Don't rely on unhealthy coping strategies (such as alcohol or fast-food diets) to get you through.

6. Do your relaxation exercises (see pp. 145–8).

7. Nourish your body and mind in equal measure.

Marguerite

I'm always careful now and try to look after my health as much as I can so I don't have setbacks. For me, it was mainly a question of learning to trust my body again. I always worry about flu season, but take special precautions. For me, forewarned is forearmed.

Julia

I haven't had any serious setbacks. Although I do sometimes overdo it when I stay up late or let my healthy habits slide.

CHAPTER THIRTEEN
CFS and Your Relationships

When someone has a brief injury or illness, there is almost always the understanding that the person will eventually bounce back and be fully functioning again. He or she might be out of commission for a time, but because the period of unwellness generally has a predictable course – start, convalescence and recovery – the process can be managed and tolerated.

With a chronic illness, however, where the outcome is unknown, the whole family suffers too. Adjustments have to be made, lifestyle standards are often reduced and everyone's life is affected. The process of adjustment with CFS can be particularly chaotic and unsettling since the course of the illness is often physically and emotionally uncertain.

Sometimes, for weeks, months or even years, you may feel well, almost normal. The whole family then breathes a sigh of relief, until a viral infection or other setback occurs, and then it is back to square one. Some days, you might be fully or nearly independent – walking, washing, driving – but the very next, you are barely able to get out of bed. CFS is a rollercoaster of every physical and psychological dimension. And it is hard to take each day as it comes, when so much of life – work, bills, mortgages, schooling, meal preparation – requires certainty.

Added to this heady mix is the fact that as a CFS sufferer you may have had to fight hard to prove the legitimacy of your illness. Even friends and family members might struggle to accept that you are not attention seeking at times or 'putting it on' because of the mixed messages they receive from the medical community and the odd combination of the person who seems fine one day and bedridden the next.

When CFS strikes, because everyone suffers, carers can end up feeling resentful, angry, bitter and frustrated. And, as a result, you will often feel guilty. Relationships need to be strong in order to survive.

Improving Relationships

Most relationships can hit a snag from time to time. And with CFS in the equation, even the most loving and stable relationships are put to the test. In fact, it is not uncommon for marriages or partnerships to break down.[1] While denial might seem an attractive option when this starts to happen – hoping that the whole horrible business of CFS and any resulting relationship difficulties will magically go away – it's not. Tensions simmer, fuelling resentment. So the best strategy for navigating the illness is to face the problems head on, acknowledge them and work together to deal with them.

For you

CFS triggers all kinds of conflicting and unpleasant feelings which can be worrying and scary. Many sufferers try to cope with these distressing emotions on their own, while others tend to share every stressful thought and feeling because they feel isolated and unable to cope with their unbearable situation. They crave love, support, reassurance and comfort. Both strategies in the extreme can be damaging. Bottling things up leads to the stress that can further disable you; but share every gloomy sensation and you run the risk of compassion fatigue in others around you.

Striking the right balance is the key to successful communication and healthier relationships. Here are some tips to help you achieve this:

- **Maintain good communication.** This means being willing to talk openly about your own concerns but, equally, it means listening to the needs of your carers. The world of chronic illness is all consuming, not just for you, but for the other people in your life. Both you and they have a right to be scared, fed up and annoyed. But you are in this together, so try to keep up a team mentality.

- **Keep a journal** A diary is a good way to dredge up and release any built-up frustrations, worries and anxieties you might have. Here you can spill your guts out, completely freely and uninhibited, without fear of rebuke or rejection from others. If you are easily fatigued, you can keep the language very simple and don't worry about grammar.

- **Be respectful of others** Your family members might not fully understand your debilitation. They are only human. Show appreciation for their efforts, even if they are not always meeting your needs. Also, always remember to ask them about what is going on in their life.

- **Face problems as they crop up** In addition to the day-to-day grind of chronic illness, other challenges emerge: money difficulties, physical intimacy issues, child-rearing. Don't just assume that these problems will go away on their own or that other people will willingly take on the burden of handling them alone.

- **Seek outside support** Don't run the risk of alienating those in your life by draining them with all your demands. Join the local CFS support group (see Resources, p. 193). Often they can be contacted online or by phone. Even the Samaritans can provide a sympathetic ear twenty-four hours a day. And you can always contact your GP for a counselling referral.

- **Encourage others to engage in the activities they enjoy** It is not always easy to see your family or friends going out, socialising, catching the latest film release or basically enjoying life, while you are stuck indoors or in bed. However, you should actively encourage your friends and family to let off steam and enjoy themselves. Don't make them feel guilty for doing so. It is not their fault you are ill.

- **Ask for assistance** No one likes to be dependent on others, but with CFS you may need extensive care at some point in your recovery. So don't be proud. If you need help ask for it. You have an illness and a genuine need. And remember, if you exceed your capabilities, you could end up even worse and more dependent than ever.

- **Be more than your illness** CFS may dominate your life, but it is not who you are. While the condition can consume most of your thoughts and feelings, you are not just a bunch of symptoms. You are more than that. So try to take moments when you can and enjoy 'normal' life. These pleasures might be as simple as watching television, listening to the radio or even sitting downstairs with others for a while. But you will not feel so isolated.

- **Be realistic** Don't over-dramatise your symptoms. CFS is a serious problem, but try not to turn the situation into an Oscar-winning performance. You will feel miserable, but right now remember you are on the road to recovery. Having said that, don't try to play down or minimise your illness or symptoms either. That's just denial.

- **Don't expect people to be psychic** Don't assume that others will automatically know you want the window closed, the radio turned off or that you want a rest. Tell them what you need. However, you might want to be organised with your requests and try to be flexible. Make lists and prioritise. If something doesn't get done today, there is always tomorrow.

- **Inform others about CFS** You might look healthy, so many won't quite understand why you say you are so ill. The prejudices and misconceptions about the condition may take hold even within the family and among friends. Show them this book and provide factual and accurate information about Chronic Fatigue Syndrome.

- **Never take anyone for granted** Just two little words – thank you – have such magical properties because we all like to feel appreciated.

For partners and carers

CFS is a nightmare for you too. I understand this. Families, parents, friends and spouses are so often the unsung heroes in this horrific ordeal and very rarely receive due acknowledgement or appreciation for the sacrifices they make. Many also feel helpless, scared and uncertain. Roles in the family often reverse and plans are thrown out of the window as, out of the blue, long-term illness charges into their life, unwanted and uninvited.

You might have vowed for better or worse, in sickness and in health, but if your wife, husband or partner has CFS, *your* life will completely change too. Serious adjustments in terms of finances, domestic set-ups, childcare and household chores will need to be made. You will probably assume the roles of carer, sole income earner, parent and housekeeper. And all these unexpected and unanticipated stresses and strains can lead to a build-up of resentment. It might even contribute to your own emotional and physical ill health.

Here are some tips to help you cope with your changed circumstances:

- **Accept your life has changed** This is no time for denial. Without dwelling on the misery of the situation, sit down and draft a plan on how you are going to cope domestically, financially, physically and emotionally.

- **Don't be superhuman** You might want to keep everything private, assume all the responsibilities yourself and kid yourself that everything is OK. This is a mistake. Don't do it all. Delegate where you can. If everyone contributes a little, the burden can be eased.

- **Accept that the illness is genuine** This is essential. Your loved one might not look it, but they really are ill. No one would choose to be this debilitated and dependent on their families for every aspect of care.

- **Don't minimise their symptoms** It is often very difficult to understand the full extent of disability with CFS, even when you live alongside someone who has it. You might feel tired too, say after a hard day's work, but the exhaustion that someone with CFS feels is off the scale. When carers, sometimes even well-meaning ones, minimise the extent of debilitation, this leads to guilt on the part of the patient and can force them to do more than they are able.

- **Seek support yourself** Instead of letting frustrations build up, only to explode at some point, or isolating yourself in a world of illness, remember you are human and you need to offload too. Talk to your doctor about a local carers' group or start one up yourself. You might also want to speak to a counsellor or therapist to help you cope with feelings of anger and resentment and the veritable tsunami of changes you and your family are now forced to face. You too have needs and must address them.

- **Look after your health** This is obvious. If you go down, they all go down with you.

- **Remind yourself that your loved one is on the road to recovery** It might take hard work and a ton of patience, but others have reached their goal and your partner will too.

- **Don't assume the roles of therapist or doctor** This will only lead to frustrations. You know the patient best of all. However, you must know and accept your limitations.

Talking to Your Children

As a parent, it will be difficult to accept a diminished role in child-rearing. At this point in your recovery, you might not have the strength to participate fully in their lives and this will be upsetting for you, but equally painful for them. Children, even adult children, want Mum and Dad to be strong parental figures. So accept and expect that this is not an easy road for them either. Here are some tips to help you with this:

- **Children don't want to be different** Your illness, your diminished participation in their life and your limitations mean they will be different. They might have to be relied on as part-time or even full-time carers and this will restrict their activities, education, friendships and social life – they might not want or be able to have friends round because of your illness. So be mindful (without feeling guilty) that CFS impacts on them too.

- **Be open about your illness** Honesty is the best policy when it comes to CFS and children. It is every parent's instinct to want to protect their children from misfortune, but they have a right to know. Make sure you give them age-appropriate information and try to keep the details as simple as possible. You don't want to scare them. You can say, for example, 'I have an illness called CFS which makes me very weak and tired, but I am now working towards regaining my health'.

- **Teach your children about CFS** Encourage your children to ask you questions and explain to them the kind of symptoms you have. Tell them the reasons why you sleep during the day or feel weepy or struggle to remember things or can no longer kick a ball around the garden. Explain that these symptoms are due to the illness, *not* because you don't love them.

- **Recognise their feelings** Your child will feel angry, distressed, annoyed, afraid – in fact, all the same emotions you feel. But they might not be able to articulate them as succinctly as adults, so look for sleepless nights, bedwetting, tantrums, regressive behaviours, even denial, while they struggle to cope with your illness. Also, reassure them that you are doing everything possible to get better, even if it takes some time. Always, always, reassure them that this is not their fault.

- **Encourage them to lead a full life** Children can be very protective of their parents and they might even feel guilty if they want to go out and play or have sleepovers with their friends. Reassure them it is OK to have fun and make sure they know that you genuinely want them to enjoy themselves.

In everyday life, good communication is the best strategy for making sure everything runs as smoothly as possible. Is it perfect? No. But everyone singing from the same hymn sheet is essential during recovery, and will make you all happier and less tense along the way.

Marguerite

There are so many hardships that come with CFS, but the biggest by far has to be my relationship with my family. It is not that they think I am faking it. Not really. But somehow, no matter how hard I tried, I could never quite convince them that I was unwell. They changed the subject or their eyes would glaze over or they would tell me to stop moaning. I would only become more upset. I finally had to accept that their sympathy pool was drained and that I would have to learn to communicate with them completely differently.

I started by showing my appreciation more and asked them more about their lives. And instead I found support through my local ME group. This was a great source of comfort to me. They knew exactly what I was going through and they became my main source of support. My home life improved dramatically.

Julia

For me, my memory was my big problem and this affected all my social relationships. I was forgetful. I couldn't keep up in conversations. My head was a jumble most of the time. People thought I was a real space case. I'd always tried to hide my illness from my friends, although my family knew. CFS has such a bad reputation, so I didn't know how others would respond and usually it was easier not to get too involved with people. I became really isolated and so lonely.

A big breakthrough came for me when I told an acquaintance I had CFS. I told her I was recovering, but sometimes my brain would get foggy. She was really kind and it was a big breakthrough for me. So I started opening up a little more, trusting people a little more. I think it helped the others too to realise the reasons why I behaved the way I did. It was a relief really because I was no longer seen as odd.

Saying Goodbye to CFS

This book is now coming to a close. Hopefully, you will have put into practice the advice here or, at the very least, have taken the information on board to learn more about your illness. Either way, I wish you well with your recovery and your plans for a healthy life.

I'm going to share with you now one final useful technique that I routinely use with my patients: saying goodbye to CFS in a letter. This illness was an unwanted companion in your life and its impact will have been severe. As you make the transition from patient to healthy person, leaving behind the life of an invalid, I want you to jot down your feelings: what you've learned about yourself, the inner strengths you never knew you had, the lows, the highs, the good, the bad, the ugly. Next, write down all your hopes for the future, your plans, your dreams, your goals. Finally, say goodbye to CFS.

The letter is for your eyes only, so there's no need to worry about grammar or making it perfect. Once you've finished, put it away in a drawer and in a month's time – not before – take it out and reread it. Your written words will help to focus your thoughts and remind you of the incredible challenge you have been forced to face. Keep the letter handy for whenever you need a morale boost. You've achieved the near impossible. You've survived CFS! You should be proud of yourself. Go out now and live a life of joy.

Depression Mimickers

As we have already seen, depression can reflect a number of processes that malfunction in CFS. Also, as with CFS, depression can have a number of mimickers.

Here are some of the more common conditions often mistaken for depression:

Neurological

- Dementia
- Epilepsy
- Fahr's syndrome
- Huntington's disease
- Infections
- Migraines
- Multiple sclerosis
- Narcolepsy
- Parkinson's disease
- Stroke

Endocrinal

- Adrenal (Cushing's, Addison's) disease
- Hyperthyroidism
- Hypothyroidism
- Menses-related problems
- Parathyroid disorders
- Post-partum complications

Infectious and inflammatory

- AIDS
- Bacterial pneumonia
- Lupus
- Mononucleosis/glandular fever
- Rheumatoid arthritis
- Sjögren's syndrome
- Temporal arthritis
- Tuberculosis
- Viral pneumonia

Miscellaneous

- Cancer (especially pancreatic and stomach)
- Cardiopulmonary disease
- Porphyria
- Vitamin deficiencies (such as B^{12}, C, folate, niacin and thiamine)

And the following drugs can also be culprits:

Analgesic and anti-inflammatory drugs

- Ibuprofen
- Indomethacin
- Opiates
- Phenacetin
- Ampicillin
- Cycloserine
- Ethionamide
- Metronidazole

- Nalidixic acid
- Nitrofurantoin
- Streptomycin
- Sulfamethoxazole
- Sulfanomides
- Tetracycline

Blood pressure/cardiac drugs

- Alphamethldopa
- Beta blockers
- Bethanidine
- Clonidine
- Digitalis
- Guanethidine
- Hydralazine
- Lidocaine
- Methoserpidine
- Prazosin
- Procainamide
- Quanabenzacetate
- Rescinnamine
- Reserpine
- Veratrum

Neurological and psychiatric drugs

- Almantadine
- Baclofen
- Bromocriptine
- Carbamazepine
- Levodopa
- Neuroleptics
- Phenytoin
- Sedatives
- Tetrabenazine

Steroids and hormones

- Corticosteroids
- Danazol
- Oral contraceptives
- Prednisone
- Triamcinolone

Recreational substances

- Alcohol
- Methadone
- Heroin
- Sedatives
- Cocaine/crack cocaine
- Ecstasy
- Marijuana
- PCP

This list is not exhaustive – if you can believe it! The medical and pharmaceutical conditions that produce depressive symptoms, irrespective of brain chemical malfunctions or stressful life events, are virtually endless. If you are on certain medications or have been diagnosed with some other illness, then secondary depression cannot be ignored as a potential source of mood deterioration.

The Big Five Exercise – the Answers

Here are the answers to the big five exercise on p. 118 (1, 2 and 3 were already supplied):

4. Physiology
5. Environment
6. Emotion
7. Environment
8. Physiology
9. Thought
10. Environment
11. Environment
12. Emotion
13. Physiology
14. Thought
15. Environment
16. Emotion
17. Emotion
18. Emotion
19. Environment
20. Environment
21. Environment
22. Physiology
23. Physiology

24. Thought
25. Emotion
26. Physiology
27. Thought
28. Emotion
29. Thought
30. Physiology
31. Behaviour
32. Behaviour
33. Thought
34. Emotion
35. Behaviour
36. Behaviour
37. Emotion
38. Behaviour
39. Behaviour
40. Physiology

Resources

Key Contacts and Support Groups

United Kingdom

Action for M.E.
PO Box 2778
Bristol BS21 9DJ
Tel.: 0845 123 2380/0117 927 9551
Email: admin@afme.org.uk
www.afme.org.uk

The ME Association
7 Apollo Office Court
Radclive Road
Gawcott
Bucks MK18 4DF
Tel: 01200 010964
Email: meconnect@meassociation.org.uk
www.meassociation.org.uk

The National M.E. Centre and Centre for Fatigue Syndromes
National ME Centre
Disablement Services Centre
Old Harold Wood Hospital Site
Harold Wood
Romford
Essex RM3 0BE
Tel.: 01708 378050
Email: nmecent@aol.com
www.nmec.org.uk

Dr Kristina Downing-Orr
76 Harley Street Clinic
London W1G 7HH
Tel. 020 7631 3276
www.76HarleyStreet.com

Alessandro Ferretti and Jules Cattell
Equilibria Health
Elmcroft
Dorsington
Warwickshire CV37 8AT
Tel.: 0845 620 9718/01789 778834
Email: info@equilibria-health.co.uk
www.equilibria-health.co.uk

Alessandro Ferretti and Jules Cattell
76 Harley Street
London W1G 7HH
Tel.: 020 7631 3276
www.76HarleyStreet.com

Dr David Mason Brown
Medical Director
In Equilibrium
1 Hillpark Crescent
Edinburgh
Midlothian EH4 7BG
Tel.: 0131 476 7183
www.cfs-me.co.uk
www.in-equilibrium.co.uk

Irish Republic

Irish ME/CFS Association
PO Box 3075
Dublin 2
Tel.: 01 235 0965
Email: info@irishmecfs.org
www.irishmecfs.org

USA and Canada

CFIDS Association of America
PO Box 220398
Charlotte, NC 28222–0398
Tel.: (704) 365 2343
Email: cfids@cfids.org
www.cfids.org

International Association for
Chronic Fatigue Syndrome/ME
27 N Wacker Drive Suite 416
Chicago, IL 60606
Tel.: (847) 258 7248
Email: Admin@iacfsme.org
www.iacfs.net

National Fibromyalgia Association
2121 S. Towne Centre Place
Suite 300
Anaheim, CA 92806
Tel.: (714) 921 0150
www.fmaware.org

National Chronic Fatigue and Immune
Dysfunction Syndrome Association
103 Aletha Road
Needham, MA 02492
Tel.: (781) 449 3535
Email: info@ncf.net.org
www.ncf-net.org

Fibromyalgia Network
PO 31750
Tucson, AZ 85751–1750
Tel.: (800) 853 2929
Email: inquiry@fmnetnews.com
www.fmnetnews.com

Myalgic Encephalitis Association of Ontario
Ste. 402, 170 Donway West
Toronto ON M3C 2G3
Tel.: (416) 222 8820
Email: info@meao-cfs.on.ca
http://meao.ca

Nightingale Research Foundation
121 Iona Street
Ottawa
Ontario K1Y 3M1
Tel.: (613) 523 1958
Email: info@nightingale.ca
www.nightingale.ca

Australia

ME/CFS Australia
PO Box 7100
Dandenong Vic 3175
Tel.: 039793 4500
Email: ceo@mecfs.org.au
www.MECFS.org.au

ME/CFS Society of NSW
PO Box 5403
West Chatswood
NSW 1515
Tel.: (02) 9904 8433
Email mesoc@zip.com.au
www.me-cfs.org.au

ME/CFS Australia (Northern Territory)
GPO Box 1363
Darwin NT 0801
Tel.: (08) 8941 2635
Email: admin@mecfs-nt.org.au
www.me-cfs.nt.org.au

ME/CFS/FM Support Association Qld Inc.
CIO Mission Department
St. Vincent Hopital, Scott Street
Toowoomba
QLD 4350
Tel.: (07) 4632 8173
Email: mefmtba@bigpond.com
www.mecfsfmq.org.au

ME/CFS Australia (South Australia) Inc.
GPO Box 383
Adelaide, SA 5001
Tel.: (08) 8410 8299
Email: sacfs@sacfs.asn.au
www.sacfs.asn.au

ME/CFS Australia (Victoria)
PO Box 7100
DANDENONG VIC 3175
Tel.: (03) 9791 2199
Email: admin@mecfs-vic.org.au
www.mecfs-vic.org.au

New Zealand

Associated NZ Myalgic Encephalopathy Society
PO Box 36–307
Northcote
Auckland NZ
Tel.: (09) 269 6374
Email: info@anzmes.org.nz
http://www.anzmes.org.nz

South Africa

MEASA (ME Association of South Africa)
PO Box 1802
Umhlanga Rocks
4320
South Africa
Email: arl@telkomsa.net
http://www.me.org.za

Stockists for Vitamin and Mineral Supplements

Arkopharma UK Ltd
7 Redlands Centre
Coulsdon
Surrey CR5 2HT
Tel.: 020 8763 1414
Email: sales@arkopharma.co.uk
www.arkopharma.com

BioCare, Lakeside
180 Lifford Lane
Kings Norton
Birmingham B30 3NU
Tel.: 0121 433 3727

Email: biocare@biocare.co.uk
www.biocare.co.uk

Blackmores Australia
20 Jubilee Avenue
Warriewood NSW 2102
Tel.: 61 2 9910 5000
www.blackmores.com.au

Blackmores New Zealand
API Consumer Brands Ltd
14–16 Norman Spencer Drive
Manukau City
Auckland NZ
Tel.: (64) 9279 7979
Email: customerservices@api.net.nz
www.blackmoresnz.co.nz

G + G Vitamins
2/3 Imberhorne Way
East Grinstead
West Sussex, RH19 IRL
Tel.: (0) 1342 312811
www.gandgvitamins.com
sales@gandgvitamins.com

Holland & Barrett
Samuel Ryder House
Barling Way
Eliot Park
Nuneaton
Warwickshire CV10 7RH
Tel.: 0870 606 6605
Email: healthinformation@hollandandbarrett.com
www.hollandandbarrett.com

Prime Directive – Safe Remedies
Unit 11
Windmill Way West
Ramparts Business Park
Berwick-Upon-Tweed TD15 1TB
Tel.: 01289 332 888
www.saferemedies.com

Solgar Vitamins Ltd
Aldbury, Tring,
Hertfordshire HP23 5PT
Tel.: 01442 890 355
www.solgar.co.uk

Solgar New Zealand
PO Box 12546
Penrose, Auckland
New Zealand
Tel.: (09) 525 2355
Email: sales@solgar.co.nz
www.solgar.com

Solgar South Africa
PO Box 1217
Northriding 2162
South Africa
Tel.: (27) 11 462 1652
Email: infosa@solgar.com
www.solgar.com

References

Meet the Experts

1. Mason Brown, D., personal communication.
2. Ferretti, A., personal communication.

Introduction

1. Gelder, M. et al., *The Shorter Oxford Textbook of Psychiatry* (5th edition), OUP Oxford, 2006; Lisman, S. R. and Dougherty, K., *Chronic Fatigue Syndrome for Dummies*, John Wiley & Sons, 2007; Puri, B. K., *Chronic Fatigue Syndrome: A Natural Way to Treat M.E.*, Hammersmith Press Limited, 2004; Shepherd, C., *Living with M.E.: The Chronic/ Post-viral Fatigue Syndrome*, Vermilion, 1999.
2. Gelder, M. et al., *The Shorter Oxford Textbook of Psychiatry* (5th edition), OUP Oxford, 2006.
3. Ibid.
4. Burgess, M. and Chalder, T., *Overcoming Chronic Fatigue: A Self-help Guide Using Cognitive Behavioural Techniques*, Robinson Publishing, 2005; Chalder, T., *Coping with Chronic Fatigue (Overcoming Common Problems)*, Seldon Press, 1995.
5. The *Psychologist*, June 2009, vol. 33, no. 63, pp.256–64.
6. MacIntyre, A., *M.E./Chronic Fatigue Syndrome: A Practical Guide*, Thorsons, 1991; Mason Brown, D., personal communication; Shepherd, C., op. cit.
7. Lisman, S. R. and Dougherty, K., op. cit.; Puri, B. K. op. cit.; Shepherd, C., op. cit.
8. Mason Brown, D., personal communication.

9. Downing-Orr, K., *Rethinking Depression: Why Current Treatments Fail*, Plenum, 1998; Downing-Orr, K., *What to Do if You're Burned Out and Blue*, Thorsons, 2000.

Chapter One

1. Lisman, S. R. and Dougherty, K., *Chronic Fatigue Syndrome for Dummies*, John Wiley & Sons, 2007.
2. Mason Brown, D., personal communication.
3. Courmel, K., *A Companion Volume to Dr. Jay A. Goldstein's Betrayal by the Brain: A Guide for Patients and Their Physicians*, Haworth Medical Press Inc., 1996; MacIntyre, A., *M.E./Chronic Fatigue Syndrome: A Practical Guide*, Thorsons, 1991; Mason Brown, D., personal communication; Puri, B. K., *Chronic Fatigue Syndrome: A Natural Way to Treat M.E.*, Hammersmith Press Limited, 2004; Shepherd, C., *Living with M.E.: The Chronic/Post-viral Fatigue Syndrome*, Vermilion, 1999; Shepherd, C. and Chauduri, A., *ME/CFS/PVFS: An Exploration of the Key Clinical Issues* (3rd edition), The ME Association, 2007; Teitelbaum, J., *From Fatigued to Fantastic*, Avery Publishing Group, 2007.
4. Shepherd, C. and Chauduri, A., op. cit.
5. Puri, B. K., op. cit.
6. Ibid.
7. Lisman, S. R. and Dougherty, K., op. cit.
8. Lisman, S. R. and Dougherty, K., op. cit.; MacIntyre, A., op. cit.; Shepherd, C., op. cit.
9. Shepherd, C., op. cit.
10. MacIntyre, A., op. cit.; Lisman, S. R. and Dougherty, K., op. cit.; Shepherd, C., op. cit.
11. Kerr, J. et al., 'Microbial infections in eight genomic subtypes of chronic fatigue syndrome/myalgic enceophalomyelitis', *Journal of Clinical Pathology*, 2010, 63, pp. 156–64.

Chapter Two

1. Carruthers, B. M. and van de Sande, M. I., 'Myalgic Encephalomyelitis/Chronic Fatigue Syndrome: A Clinical Case Definition and Guidelines for Medical Practitioners', an overview of the Canadian Consensus document, ISBN 0-9739335-O-X, 2005.
2. Shepherd, C., *Living with M.E.: The Chronic/Post-viral Fatigue Syndrome*, Vermilion, 1999.
3. De Meirleir, K. V. and Englebienne, P., *Chronic Fatigue Syndrome: A Biological Approach*, CRC Press, 2002.
4. Teitelbaum, J., *From Fatigued to Fantastic*, Avery Publishing Group, 2007.
5. Shepherd, C., op. cit.; Teitelbaum, J., op. cit.
6. Carruthers, B. M. and van de Sande, S. I., op. cit.
7. Shepherd, C., op. cit., p. 32.

Chapter Three

1. Teitelbaum, J., *From Fatigued to Fantastic*, Avery Publishing Group, 2007.
2. Ali, M., 2003, 'The cause of Fibro Myalgia: the respiratory-to-fermentative shift (the Dysox State) in ATP production', *Journal of Integrative Medicine* 8: p. 140; Buskila, D. and Newman, L., 2005, 'Genetics of Fibro Myalgia', Current Pain and Headache Reports, 9 (5), pp. 313–15.
3. Downing-Orr, K., *Rethinking Depression: Why Current Treatments Fail*, Plenum, 1998; Downing-Orr, K., *What to Do if You're Burned Out and Blue*, Thorsons, 2000.
4. Ibid.

Chapter Four

1. McEvedy, C. P. and Beard, A. W., 'Royal Free epidemic of 1955 – A Reconsideration', *British Medical Journal*, 1970, 1, pp. 7–11.
2. Mason Brown, D., personal communication; Twisk, Frank N. M. and Maes, Michael, 2009, 'A review on cognitive behavioural therapy (CBT) and graded exercise therapy (GET) in myalgic encephalomyelitis (ME)/ chronic fatigue syndrome (CFS): CBT/GET is not only ineffective and not evidence-based, but also potentially harmful for many patients with ME/CF', *Neuroendocrinology Letters*, Volume 30, No. 3, pp. 284–99.
3. Gelder, M. et al., *The Shorter Oxford Textbook of Psychiatry* (5th edition), OUP Oxford, 2006.
4. Friedberg, F. and Sohl, S., 'Cognitive behavioural therapy in chronic fatigue syndrome: Is improvement related to increased physical activity?' *Journal of Clinical Psychology*, 2009, Vol. 65, pp. 1–20.

Chapter Five

1. Puri, B. K., *Chronic Fatigue Syndrome: A Natural Way to Treat M.E.*, Hammersmith Press Limited, 2004; Shepherd, C., *Living with M.E.: The Chronic/Post-viral Fatigue Syndrome*, Vermilion, 1999; Mason Brown, D., personal communication.
2. Shepherd, C., op. cit.; MacIntyre, A., *M.E./Chronic Fatigue Syndrome: A Practical Guide*, Thorsons, 1991.
3. Shepherd, C., op. cit.
4. Lisman, S. R. and Dougherty, K., *Chronic Fatigue Syndrome for Dummies*, John Wiley & Sons, 2007; Shepherd, C., op. cit.
5. Shepherd, C., op. cit; MacIntyre, A., op. cit.; Mason Brown, D., personal communication.
6. Lisman, S. R. and Dougherty, K., op. cit.; MacIntyre, A., op. cit.; Mason Brown, D., personal communication; Shepherd, C. and Chauduri, A., *ME/CFS/PVFS: An Exploration of the*

Key Clinical Issues (3rd edition), The ME Association, 2007; Shepherd, C., op. cit.

7. Burgess, M. and Chalder. T., *Overcoming Chronic Fatigue: A Self-help Guide Using Cognitive Behavioural Techniques*, Robinson Publishing, 2005.
8. BBC News at One, Friday, 9 October 2009.
9. Shepherd, C., op. cit.
10. Lisman, S. R. and Dougherty, K., op. cit.; Mason Brown, D., personal communication; Shepherd, C., op. cit.
11. Dr Gwen Sprehn, 'Decreased cancer survival in individuals separated at time of diagnosis: critical period for pathophysiology', *Cancer*, 2009, vol. 115, issue 21, pp. 5108–16.
12. Shepherd, C., op. cit.; Teitelbaum, J., *From Fatigued to Fantastic*, Avery Publishing Group, 2007; MacIntyre, A., op. cit.; Puri, B. K., op. cit.
13. Puri, B. K., op. cit.; Shepherd, C., op. cit.
14. Ibid.
15. Puri, B. K., op. cit.
16. Shepherd, C., op. cit.; Teitelbaum, J., op. cit.
17. Shepherd, C., op. cit.
18. Mason Brown, D., personal communication.
19. Mason Brown, D., personal communication; Teitelbaum, J., op. cit.

Chapter Seven

1. MacIntyre, A., *M.E./Chronic Fatigue Syndrome: A practical guide*, Thorsons, 1991; Shepherd, C., *Living with M.E.: The Chronic/Post-viral Fatigue Syndrome*, Vermilion, 1999.
2. Mason Brown, D., personal communication.

Chapter Twelve

1. MacIntyre, A., *M.E./Chronic Fatigue Syndrome: A Practical Guide*, Thorsons, 1991; Mason Brown, D., personal communication;

Shepherd, C., *Living with M.E.: The Chronic/Post-viral Fatigue Syndrome*, Vermilion, 1999.

Chapter Thirteen

1. Mason Brown, D., personal communication.

Bibliography

Primary Sources

This work is original and based largely on primary sources. My own personal experiences of CFS, my qualifications in clinical psychology, CBT and NLP, my daily tutorials with Dr Mason Brown and in-depth discussions with fellow CFS patients formed the basis for my research on this book. The ME Association and Action for ME in Britain also supplied essential information.

Secondary Sources

I also consulted the following secondary sources in researching this book:

Akagi, H., et al., 'Cognitive behaviour therapy for chronic fatigue syndrome in a general hospital – feasible and effective', *General Hospital Psychiatry*, 2001, vol. 23, issue 5, pp. 254–60.

Appel. S., et al., 'Infection and vaccination in chronic fatigue syndrome: Myth or reality?', *Autoimmunity*, 2007, vol. 40, no.1, pp. 48–53.

Armitage, R. et al., 'The impact of a 4-hour sleep delay on slow-wave activity in twins discordant for chronic fatigue syndrome', *Sleep*, 2007, vol. 30, issue 5, pp. 657–62.

Ayres, J. G., et al., 'Post-infection fatigue syndrome following Q fever', *Quarterly Journal of Medicine*, 1998, vol. 91, issue 2, pp. 105–23.

Bazelmans, E., et al., 'Is physical deconditioning a perpetuating factor in chronic fatigue syndrome? A controlled study on maximal exercise performance and relations with fatigue, impairment and physical activity', *Psychological Medicine*, 2001, vol. 31, issue 1, pp. 107–14.

Behan, W. M. H., et al., 'Mitochondrial abnormalities in the postviral fatigue syndrome', *Acta Neurologica Scandinavica*, 1991, vol. 83, no. 1, pp. 61–5.

Black, C. D., et al., 'Increased daily physical activity and fatigue symptoms in chronic fatigue syndrome', *Dynamic Medicine*, 2005, 4:3.

Bou-Holaigah, I., et al., 'The relationship between neurally mediated hypotension and the chronic fatigue syndrome', *Journal of the American Medical Association*, 1995, vol. 274, no. 12, pp. 961–7.

Buchwald, D., et al., 'A chronic illness characterized by fatigue, neurologic and immunological disorders, and active human herpes type 6 infection', *Annals of Internal Medicine*, 1992, vol. 116, issue 2, pp. 103–13.

Buchwald, D., et al., 'Functional status in patients with chronic fatigue syndrome, and other fatiguing illnesses, and healthy individuals', *American Journal of Medicine*, 1996, vol. 101, issue 4, pp. 36–370.

Buchwald, D., et al., 'A twin study of chronic fatigue syndrome', *Psychosomatic Medicine*, 2001, 63, 936–43.

Cameron, B., et al., 'Prolonged illness after infectious mononucleosis is associated with altered immunity but not with increased viral load', *Journal of Infectious Diseases*, 2006, vol. 193, no. 5 pp. 664–71.

Deale, A. and Wessely, S., 'Diagnosis of psychiatric disorder in clinical evaluation of chronic fatigue syndrome', *Journal of the Royal Society of Medicine*, 2000, vol. 93, issue 6, pp. 310–12.

Deale, A., et al., 'Cognitive behaviour therapy for the chronic fatigue syndrome: a randomised controlled trial', *American Journal of Psychiatry*, 1997, vol. 154, issue 3, pp. 408–14.

Deale, A., et al., 'Illness beliefs and outcomes in chronic fatigue syndrome: do patients need to change their beliefs in order to get better?', *Journal of Psychosomatic Research*, 1998, vol. 45, issue 1, pp. 77–83.

Deale, A. et al., 'Long-term outcome of cognitive behaviour therapy versus relaxation therapy for chronic fatigue syndrome: a 5-year follow-up study', *American Journal of Psychiatry*, 2001, vol. 158, issue 12, pp. 2038–42.

de Lange, F. P., et al., 'Neural correlates of the chronic fatigue syndrome', *Brain*, 2004, vol. 127, no. 9, pp. 1948–9.

de Lange, F. P., et al., 'Gray matter volume reduction in the chronic fatigue syndrome', *Neuroimage*, 2005, vol. 26, issue 3, pp. 777–81.

de Luca, J., et al., 'Cognitive functioning is impaired in patients with chronic fatigue syndrome devoid of psychiatric disease', *Journal of Neurology, Neurosurgery and Psychiatry*, 1997, vol. 62, pp. 151–5.

Demitrack, M. E., et al., 'Evidence for impaired activation of the hypothalamic-pituitary-adrenal axis in patients with chronic fatigue syndrome', *Journal of Clinical Endocrinology and Metabolism*, 1991, vol. 73, no. 6, pp. 1224–34.

Diaz-Mitoma, F., et al., 'Clinical improvement in chronic fatigue syndrome is associated with enhanced natural killer cell-mediated cytotoxicity: the results of a pilot study with isoprinosine', *Journal of Chronic Fatigue Syndrome*, 2003, vol. 11, issue 2, pp. 71–95.

Dismukes, W. E., et al., 'A randomised, double-blind trial of Nystatin therapy for the candidasis hypersensitivity syndrome', *New England Journal of Medicine*, 1990, vol. 323, no. 25, pp. 1717–23.

Farmer, A., et al., 'Screening for psychiatric morbidity in subjects presenting with chronic fatigue syndrome', *British Journal of Psychiatry*, 1996, vol. 168, pp. 354–8.

Faulkner, S. and Smith, A., 'A longitudinal study of the relationship between psychological distress and recurrence of upper-respiratory tract infections in chronic fatigue syndrome', *British Journal of Health Psychology*, 18 December 2006 [Epub ahead of print].

Freeman, R. and Komaroff A. L., 'Does the chronic fatigue syndrome involve the autonomic nervous system?', *American Journal of Medicine*, 1997, vol. 102, issue 4, pp. 357–64.

Freeman, R., 'The chronic fatigue syndrome is a disease of the autonomic nervous system. Sometimes', *Clinical Autonomic Research*, 2002, vol. 12, no. 4, pp. 231–3.

Friedberg, F. and Krupp, L. B., 'A comparison of cognitive

behavioural treatment for chronic fatigue syndrome and primary depression', *Clinical Infectious Diseases*, 1994, 18 (suppl. 1), S105–10.

Fukuda, K., et al., 'The chronic fatigue syndrome. A comprehensive approach to its definition and study', *Annals of Internal Medicine*, 1994, 121, pp. 953–9.

Fulcher, K. Y. and White, P. D., 'Randomised controlled trial of graded exercise in patients with chronic fatigue syndrome', *British Medical Journal*, 1997, vol. 314, pp. 1647–52.

Georgiades, E., et al., 'Chronic fatigue syndrome: new evidence for a central fatigue disorder', *Clinical Science*, 2003, vol. 105, no. 2, pp. 213–18.

Gow, J. W., et al., 'Antiviral pathway activation in patients with chronic fatigue syndrome and acute infection', *Clinical Infectious Diseases*, 2001, vol. 33, pp. 2080–1.

Grans, H., et al., 'Gene expression profiling in the chronic fatigue syndrome', *Journal of Internal Medicine*, 2005, vol. 258, issue 4, pp. 288–390.

Hinds, G. M. E., et al., 'A retrospective study of the chronic fatigue syndrome', *Proceedings of the Royal College of Physicians of Edinburgh*, 1993, 23, pp. 10–14.

Huibers, M. J., et al., 'Efficacy of cognitive-behavioural therapy by general practitioners for unexplained fatigue among employees : randomised controlled trial', *British Journal of Psychiatry*, 2004, vol. 184, issue 3, pp. 240–6.

Hurel, S. J., et al., 'Patients with a self-diagnosis of myalgic encephalomyelitis', *British Medical Journal*, 1995, vol. 311, p. 329.

Keenan, P. A., 'Brain MRI abnormalities exist in chronic fatigue syndrome', *Journal of Neurological Sciences*, 1999, vol. 172, issue 1, pp. 1–2.

Lane, R. J. M., 'Chronic fatigue syndrome: is it physical?', *Journal of Neurology, Neurosurgery and Psychiatry*, 2000, vol. 69, issue 3, p. 280.

Lapp, C. W., 'Exercise limits in the chronic fatigue syndrome', *American Journal of Medicine*, 1997, vol. 103, issue 1, pp. 83–4.

Lloyd, A. R., et al., 'Immunologic and psychological therapy for patients with chronic fatigue syndrome: a double-blind, placebo-controlled trial', *American Journal of Medicine*, 1993, vol. 94, pp. 197–203.

Lyall, M., et al., 'A systematic review and critical evaluation of the immunology of chronic fatigue syndrome', *Journal of Psychosomatic Research*, 2003, vol. 55, issue 2, pp. 79–90.

McCully, K. and Natelson, B. H., 'Impaired oxygen delivery to muscle in chronic fatigue syndrome', *Clinical Science*, 1999, vol. 97, no. 5, pp. 603–8.

Michiels, V. and Cluydts, R., 'Neuropsychological functioning in chronic fatigue syndrome', *Acta Psychiatrica Scandinavica*, 2001, vol. 103, issue 2, pp. 84–93.

Moldofsky, H., 'Non-restorative sleep and symptoms after a febrile illness in patients with fibrositis and chronic fatigue syndromes', *Journal of Rheumatology*, 1989 (suppl. 19), 16, pp. 150–3.

Moss-Morris, R., et al., 'A randomised controlled graded exercise trial for chronic fatigue syndrome: outcomes and mechanisms for change', *Journal of Health Psychology*, 2005, vol. 10, no. 2, pp. 245–59.

Newton, J. L., et al., 'Symptoms of autonomic dysfunction in chronic fatigue syndrome', *Quarterly Journal of Medicine*, 2007, vol. 100, no. 8, pp. 519–26.

O'Dowd, H., et al., 'Cognitive behavioural therapy in chronic fatigue syndrome: a randomised controlled trial of an outpatient group programme', *Health Technology Assessment*, 2006, Oct 10 (37): iii–iv, ix–x, 1–121.

Paul, L., et al., 'Demonstration of delayed recovery from fatiguing exercise in chronic fatigue syndrome', *European Journal of Neurology*, 1999, vol. 6, pp. 63–9.

Powell, P., et al., 'Randomised controlled trial of patient education to encourage graded exercise in chronic fatigue syndrome', *British Medical Journal*, 2001, vol. 322, pp. 38–90.

Prins, J. B., et al., 'Cognitive behavioural therapy for chronic fatigue syndrome : a multicentre randomised controlled trial', *Lancet*, 2001, vol. 357, issue 9259, pp. 841–7.

Ridsdale, L., et al., 'Chronic fatigue in general practice: is counselling as good as cognitive behaviour therapy? A UK randomised trial', *British Journal of General Practice*, 2001, vol. 51, pp. 19–24.

Schweitzer, R., et al., 'Quality of life in chronic fatigue syndrome', *Social Science Medicine*, 1995, vol. 41, issue 10, pp. 1367–72.

Sharpe, M., et al., 'Cognitive behavioural therapy for chronic fatigue syndrome: a randomised controlled trial', *British Medical Journal*, 1996, vol. 312, pp. 22–6.

Sharpe, M., et al., 'Follow up of patients presenting with fatigue to an infectious diseases clinic', *British Medical Journal*, 1992, vol. 305, pp. 147–52.

Shepherd, C. B., 'Pacing and exercise in chronic fatigue syndrome', *Physiotherapy*, 2001, vol. 87, issue 8, pp. 395–6.

Straus, S. E., et al., 'Allergy and the chronic fatigue syndrome', *Journal of Allergy and Clinical Immunology*, 1988, 81, pp. 791–5.

Van Den Eede, F., et al., 'Hypothalamic-pituitary-adrenal axis function in chronic fatigue syndrome', *Neuropsychobiology*, 2007, vol. 55, issue 2, pp. 112–20.

Vercoulen, J. H. M., et al., 'Prognosis in chronic fatigue syndrome: a prospective study on the natural course', *Journal of Neurology, Neurosurgery and Psychiatry*, 1996, vol. 60, issue 5, pp. 489–94.

Vernon, S. D., et al., 'Preliminary evidence of mitochondrial dysfunction associated with post-infective fatigue after acute infection with Epstein Barr virus', *BMC Infectious Diseases*, 2006, vol. 6, p. 15.

Wallman, K. E., et al., 'Randomised controlled trial of graded exercise in chronic fatigue syndrome', *Medical Journal of Australia*, 2004, vol. 180, issue 9, pp. 444–8.

Wessely, S. and Powel, l. R., 'Fatigue syndromes: a comparison of chronic "post-viral" fatigue with neuromuscular and affective disorder', *Journal of Neurology, Neurosurgery and Psychiatry*, 1989, vol. 52, issue 8, pp. 940–8.

Yoshiuchi, K., et al., 'Patients with chronic fatigue syndrome have reduced absolute cortical blood flow', *Clinical Physiology and Functional Imaging*, 2006, vol. 26, issue 2, pp. 83–6.

Further Reading

I have included the following publications because, as well as providing research information for this book, they are also largely user-friendly. If you want to find out more about CFS or certain aspects of the illness, I would recommend any of these:

Bassman, Lynette, *The Feel-Good Guide to Fibromyalgia & Chronic Fatigue Syndrome*, New Harbinger Publications, 2007.

Bested, Alison C., Logan, Alan C. and Howe, Russell, *Hope and Help for Chronic Fatigue Syndrome and Fibromyalgia* (2nd edition), Cumberland Publications, 2008.

Burgess, Mary with Chalder, Trudie, *Overcoming Chronic Fatigue: A Self-help Guide Using Cognitive Behavioural Techniques*, Robinson Publishing, 2005.

CAM: The Magazine for Complementary and Alternative Medical Professionals, April 2008, vol. 8, issue 9.

Campbell Murdoch, Prof. J./ME Association Special Edition, *Chronic Fatigue*, Hodder & Stoughton, 2003.

Campling, Frankie and Sharpe, Michael, *Chronic Fatigue Syndrome: The Facts* (2nd edition), OUP Oxford, 2008.

Carruthers, Bruce M. and van de Sande, Marjorie I., 'Myalgic Encephalomyelitis/Chronic Fatigue Syndrome: A Clinical Case Definition and Guidelines for Medical Practitioners', an overview of the Canadian Consensus Document, Carruthers & van de Sande: Canada (ISBN: 0-9739335-O-X), 2005.

Chalder, Trudie, *Coping with Chronic Fatigue (Overcoming Common Problems)*, Seldon Press, 1995.

Courmel, Katie, *A Companion Volume to Dr. Jay A. Goldstein's Betrayal by the Brain: A Guide for Patients and Their Physicians*, Haworth Press Inc., 1996.

De Meirleir, Kenny and Englebienne, Patrick, *Chronic Fatigue Syndrome: A Biological Approach*, CRC Press, 2002.

Dilly, Susan A., Finlayson, Caroline J. and Lakhani, Sunil R., *Basic Pathology: An Introduction to the Mechanisms of Disease* (4th edition), Hodder Arnold, 2009.

Downing-Orr, Kristina, *What to do if You're Burned Out and Blue*, Thorsons, 2000.

Downing-Orr, Kristina, *Rethinking Depression: Why Current Treatments Fail*, Springer, 1998.

Downing-Orr, Kristina, *Wearing the Ruby Slippers: Nine Steps to Happiness*, Arrow Books Ltd, 2000.

Gelder, M. et al., *The Shorter Oxford Textbook of Psychiatry* (5th edition), OUP Oxford, 2006.

Goldstein, J. A., *Betrayal by the Brain: The Neurological Basis of Chronic Fatigue Syndrome, Fibromyalgia Syndrome and Related Neural Network Disorders*, Haworth Press Inc., 1997.

Holtorf, K., 'The Diagnosis and Treatment of Hypothalamic-Pituitary-Adrenal Axis Dysfunction in Patients with Chronic Fatigue Syndrome (CFS) and Fibromyalgia (FM)', *Journal of Chronic Fatigue Syndrome*, 2008, vol. 14, issue 3, pp. 59–88.

Ligman, Susan R. and Dougherty, Karla, *Chronic Fatigue Syndrome for Dummies*, John Wiley & Sons, 2007.

MacIntryre, Anne, *M.E./Chronic Fatigue Syndrome: A Practical Guide*, Thorsons, 1998.

Michell, Lynn, *Shattered: Life With M.E.*, Thorsons, 2003.

PACE trial, Patient Clinic Leaflet: 'Basic information on your illness and the treatments we can offer you for Chronic Fatigue Syndrome (CFS) also known as Myalgic Encephalomyelitis or Myalgic Encephalopathy (ME)', version 9, 5 January 2005.

Puri, Basant K., *Chronic Fatigue Syndrome: A Natural Way to Treat M.E.*, Hammersmith Press Limited, 2004.

Shepherd, Charles, *Living with M.E. The Chronic/Post-viral Fatigue Syndrome*, Vermilion, 1999.

Shepherd, Charles and Chaudhuri, Abhijit,, *ME/CFS/PVFS: An Exploration of the Key Clinical Issues* (3rd edition), The ME Association, 2007.

Staud MD, Roland and Adamec, Christine, *Fibromyalgia for Dummies*, John Wiley & Sons, 2007.

Teitelbaum, Jacob, *From Fatigued to Fantastic*, Avery Publishing Group, 2007.

White, Erica, *Erica White's Beating Fatigue Handbook*, White Publications, 2004.

While, P. D., Sharpe, M.C. and Chalder, T. 'PACE: pacing, graded activity and cognitive behavioural therapy: a randomised evaluation', information sheet, internet.

Index